Cultural Diversity, Mental Health and Psychiatry

'Black and minority ethnic communities lack confidence in mental health services', according to the *National Service Framework for Mental Health* (1999). *Cultural Diversity, Mental Health and Psychiatry* explores how and why this situation has come about, and makes specific practical, often surprising, suggestions for changing the status quo.

In his latest and most critical analysis, Suman Fernando reflects on the current situation in the light of his own personal experience, academic research and anecdotal reports. He weaves together themes of immense importance for the future of psychiatry and mental health services in a multicultural setting, exploring:

- the nature of racism and its permeation into mental health services

- the inside story of the struggle against racism in statutory and voluntary sectors of the mental health system

- the history of psychiatry and the role of spirituality, holistic thinking, psychotherapy and Asian traditions of medicine.

Trainees, practitioners and managers of mental health services will profit from the practical application of Fernando's latest ideas, and students and academics will benefit from his theoretical guidance.

Suman Fernando has been a consultant psychiatrist for over twenty years. He has written and lectured widely on mental health issues. He is Honorary Professor to the Department of Applied Social Sciences at London Metropolitan University.

Cultural Diversity, Mental Health and Psychiatry

The Struggle Against Racism

Suman Fernando

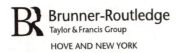

Brunner-Routledge
Taylor & Francis Group
HOVE AND NEW YORK

First published 2003 by Brunner-Routledge
27 Church Road, Hove, East Sussex, BN3 2FA

Simultaneously published in the USA and Canada
by Brunner-Routledge
29 West 35th Street, New York, NY 10001

Brunner-Routledge is an imprint of the Taylor & Francis Group

Copyright © 2003 Suman Fernando

Typeset in Times by Mayhew Typesetting, Rhayader, Powys
Printed and bound in Great Britain by TJ International Ltd,
Padstow, Cornwall
Paperback cover illustration by Jaswant Guzder
Paperback cover design by Anú Design

This publication has been produced with paper manufactured to strict
environmental standards and with pulp derived from sustainable forests.

British Library Cataloguing in Publication Data
A catalogue record for this book is available from the British Library

Library of Congress Cataloging-in-Publication Data
Fernando, Suman.
   Cultural diversity, mental health and psychiatry : the struggle
against racism / by Suman Fernando.
       p. cm.
   ISBN 1-58391-252-5 (hardback : alk. paper) — ISBN 1-58391-253-3 (pbk.:
alk. paper)
   1. Cultural psychiatry. 2. Psychiatry, Transcultural. 3. Racism. I.
Title.

   RC455.4.E8F465 2003
   362.2—dc21

                                                          2003004457

ISBN 1-58391-252-5 (hbk)
ISBN 1-58391-253-3 (pbk)

To my family in England and Sri Lanka: Frances and
Siri, Susila and Sunimal

Contents

Figure, Tables and Boxes

Figure

Tables

Boxes

Acknowledgements

I am indebted to many published works of scholarship in anthropology, psychiatry, psychology, and history. But, much more than all that I owe a great deal to a host of people who have talked to me informally over the years – people I have met as users of mental health services and professional colleagues in the mental health field in several countries, in Mind (the National Association for Mental Health in England and Wales) and the Transcultural Psychiatry Society (UK). In particular I have been influenced in my thinking by the many people I have met as workers and service users in voluntary (not-for-profit) mental health services and projects in the UK, Canada and Sri Lanka. Finally a special thanks to Jaswant Guzder who illustrated the paperback cover for this book. Jaswant Guzder is an artist, psychoanalyst and associate professor at the Division of Transcultural and Child Psychiatry, McGill University, Montreal, Canada.

Introduction

Britain is often referred to as a multicultural society, and cultural diversity is seen as a hallmark of a modern public service – be it in health, education or social care – that is equitable and open to all sections of society. Yet mental health services are frequently held to be insensitive to culture, psychiatrists and psychologists are said to be culturally incompetent and psychiatric and psychological therapies appear to be inappropriate for many people from non-western cultural backgrounds. On the one hand, much has been written that explores ways in which services may achieve cultural sensitivity or how professionals can become culturally competent; and many authorities that are responsible for delivering mental health services have policies to address race and culture, and some even have strategies to improve their services for black and other minority ethnic groups. A *national* strategy (about to be made available for consultation at the time of writing) has been drafted for this purpose within the (British) *National Service Framework for Mental Health* (Department of Health 1999). However, I have heard users of mental health services claim that services with impressive policies for cultural diversity are not necessarily any better than those without such policies; that training professionals to become culturally competent does not always mean that they treat black people any differently; that diagnoses do not make much sense, especially the diagnosis of schizophrenia; and that decision making in the allocation of therapies is often racially biased. Notwithstanding local or national strategies, a multicultural mental health service backed by a multicultural psychiatry and psychology seems to be as far off as ever. How can all this be addressed? Are the problems concerned with 'culture' or with 'race' – racism to be more exact – or with both? Have the right issues been identified and if so what attempts have been made to change things? Where do we go from here?

In 1999, the Macpherson Report (Home Department 1999) on an inquiry following a racist murder in south London made it official that public institutions in British society were institutionally racist. Some of us had been saying this for many years but the term 'institutional racism' was usually dismissed – at least in the psychiatric arena – as sociological jargon that had no practical bearing on psychiatry or the mental health services. But this is now official – the government and the opposition accept the reality of institutional racism in all public institutions, and even better, seem determined to do something about it. Since the Macpherson Report was published, I have noticed an increase in the number of conferences addressing racism in mental health services; health authorities and social service departments began allocating funds for training people to become more 'culturally sensitive' accepting that facing up to institutional racism was part and parcel of that; and even psychiatrists and psychologists began to talk about making changes in the way their successors are trained so that the next generation of professionals may be more suited to practice in a multicultural society. But I had seen something like this before in the 1980s. At that time, promoting multiculturalism was in vogue and was seen as the answer to the 'problem' that people from 'other cultures' – i.e. non-western backgrounds – were being ill served by mental health services. It struck me that nothing very much had changed as a consequence of the activities of the 1980s. I thought back to that time and the intervening twenty or so years. And I wondered how things might turn out in the future. And when I looked around, I could see debates starting again on the nature of multiculturalism and racism.

I have been involved in highlighting issues within mental health services arising from racism and cultural insensitivity for most of the past twenty years, not just at a level of individuals working in the services but at the level of institutional processes and ways of working in professional disciplines, especially psychiatry and psychology. A major problem in the mental health field has been that the main disciplines that underpin the services, namely psychiatry and psychology, have a unicultural origin – or at least they have not changed sufficiently over the years to keep up with the (cultural) changes in the composition of British society. At one time – perhaps in the late 1980s – I was optimistic that, as we came to appreciate the limitations of psychiatry and psychology arising from their ethnocentric nature and we came to understand how racism worked in the professions, especially in the way psychiatry functions as a racist system, mental health services would become 'culturally sensitive' and I even imagined that psychiatrists would be in the forefront of making the changes that were needed to bring their professional practices into the modern multicultural world. I felt that there was – and I believe that there still is – sufficient goodwill within the psychiatric profession to bring this about. In the 1980s many colleagues listened to this argument. Of course, multiculturalism was a good thing, racism has to be tackled. Genuine attempts were made to do just that although not as overtly as I would have liked.

Twenty years later when I talk, either to colleagues or at meetings, about issues around race and culture – now referred to as 'ethnic issues' – and I hear about possible ways forward, I suffer from recurrent *déjà vu*. I wonder whether we have really journeyed at all on the road or merely pretended, or perhaps just imagined that we were creating services that were sensitive to cultural differences and addressed racism. At any rate, we seem to have come back to where we started. The same topics seem to be addressed, the same wheels are being invented or perhaps now too it's all pretence.

Over the past few years I have been looking back to see what we can learn from mistakes made in the past. But at the same time I keep looking forward too. Perhaps racism and cultural diversity can be looked at from a new angle in order to explore why so little progress appears to have been made in tackling race and culture issues in psychiatry; why there has been so little change for the better in the experiences of black and Asian people who get caught up in the mental health machine – the therapies that psychiatrists and others dole out on the basis of 'knowledge' and experience. In mid-2001, I felt that the time was right for a new book since there then seemed to be a new political will to face up to institutional racism and a sense that racism is a problem for everyone, not just for black and Asian people. Since then, however, the situation has been changing; debates around multiculturalism and race have swung back 'to an altogether complacent and less challenging era' (Younge 2002: 13), and I have to take this on board.

This book is a development from themes enunciated in my earlier books, *Race and Culture in Psychiatry* (Fernando 1988) now out of print, *Mental Health, Race and Culture* (Fernando 2002) now in its second edition, and *Mental Health in a Multi-ethnic Society* (Fernando 1995a). It is about psychiatry and mental health in general and not specifically about forensic psychiatry. This is not because forensic psychiatry is not important – quite the contrary. It is in the field of forensic psychiatry that racial injustices and cultural oppression are most acutely felt by black and Asian service users. I believe that the issues in forensic psychiatry have been adequately enunciated in *Forensic Psychiatry, Race and Culture* (Fernando *et al.* 1998) and it is not necessary to repeat them here. Although my training and practical background is in psychiatry, I have been interested in the scope and practice of psychotherapy and counselling, especially since many black and Asian people look to these practices as an alternative to traditional psychiatry, when they recognise the need for help with mental health problems. I do not claim to be a psychotherapist or counsellor, nor do I claim to be particularly knowledgeable about the training of counsellors and psychotherapists. So, in addressing the field covered by these forms of 'therapy' I do so tentatively. I do not differentiate psychotherapy from counselling – both are 'talking therapies' – and I refer to the practitioners of these modes of 'therapy' as 'psychotherapists' or 'counsellors'. Finally I have not addressed issues around (language) interpreting in the fields of psychiatric counselling and psychotherapy. I believe that issues and problems encountered in using interpreters is extremely specialised and needs to be addressed by people with experience in the field. I do not claim to have any special expertise here although naturally I have used interpreters in practice.

This book is aimed at students and practitioners of psychiatry, psychology and social work, and also at people looking for academic texts; i.e. students and academics in the social sciences, especially those interested in 'race' and cultural studies and in the sociology of mental illness and health. Further, it is of relevance to managers of mental health services who have a specific duty to address race and culture issues within their services. I present several vignettes based on the narratives told to me and case histories in case notes in order to illustrate points made in the book. Although all the details are from real life, they have been combined in such a way and names of people changed so that no one person can be recognised as 'belonging' to any particular story. In other words, the stories presented are fictionalised ones of real people.

In the 1960s and 1970s, most British people of African, black Caribbean and Asian origin (black, brown and yellow people in the old-fashioned 'racial' terms) used to identify themselves, and be identified by society at large, as 'black people'. However, this began to change in the late 1980s so that now the current vogue in Britain is to refer to 'black and Asian' communities or people, rather than just 'black' communities or people. In this book, when I use the term 'black' without reference to 'Asian' or other minority ethnic communities, I do so in a political sense to refer collectively to people subjected to social and psychological exclusion from the (predominantly white) society. Yet, at the same time I adhere sometimes to the current terminology by writing of black and Asian communities or people. When reference is made to a 'struggle' or 'black struggle' (against racism), it is not to imply that black people are struggling against white people or vice versa but that there is a movement – a struggle – within society at large (and within mental health services) for human rights around (what is referred to as) 'race', akin to that in the colonial liberation movements of the 1940s and 1950s and current conflicts between the so-called 'third world' and the 'first world', for instance around migration and economic exploitation ('neo-colonialism').

In writing this book, I draw on my own and others' reflections on the issues around racism, culture and mental health, and on personal experience during a lifetime of involvement in both the statutory and voluntary sectors of the mental health field, mainly in the UK. The book falls naturally into three parts. In the first, I set the scene (background), in the second I try to explore some themes that I think are important, and in the third I try to look forward towards ways of changing practice. The background I describe is based largely on personal experience. In trying to explore why a multicultural mental health service has not got very far, I look again at racism in psychiatry. After exploring specific themes within psychiatry and psychotherapy/counselling appertaining to issues around race and culture, I attempt a brief discussion of a concept excluded from psychiatry and most forms of western psychology, namely spirituality. Then I undertake an exploration into matters around power and discrimination that underlie and promote racism through the stigma that is attached to the concept of 'mental illness' (as constructed in western culture). For this I look closely at the diagnosis of 'schizophrenia', these days almost synonymous with 'psychosis'. Essentially, I argue that psychiatric power and race power working together in combination, in collusion, is a deadly mixture. It is the custom in writing books – at least my custom – to end on a positive note however negative and pessimistic the future looks. So, in the final section of the book, I try to answer some difficult questions about the future direction of the struggle against racism in mental health services and the way forward for psychiatry if it is to become a part of this struggle rather than (as it is at present) a part of the problem we struggle against.

The book is written from a transcultural perspective that includes the view that anti-racism is part and parcel of achieving a multicultural approach. The *'Background'* to the book forms Part 1. Racism has always been a problem for black people in Britain – and there is little doubt that racism is rife on the mainland of Europe. So the vagaries of racism underlie much of the discussions in Chapter 1 (*Racism and cultural diversity*). Since the 1980s it has become increasingly obvious that the mental health services, especially the practice of psychiatry, have been problematic for black people. We have little evidence of problems around race on the mainland of Europe but I would be very surprised if they are not very similar to those in Britain. The issues were at one time referred to as issues of race and culture but are now generally referred to as 'ethnic issues'. The primary aim of this first chapter is to present these issues, but in order to do so in a way that carries some meaning of the underlying conditions, I shall consider the nature of racism as it applies in the British scene and in Europe and concepts around multiculturalism and ethnicity. The discussion of ethnic issues too would focus on British society mainly, but refer to the European scene. Finally this chapter will examine some problems in the field of psychiatric research in connection with ethnicity, race and culture.

Chapter 2 is headed *Responding to racism, addressing culture*. I start by outlining the general struggle against racism as I see it and then turn to consider the struggle in the mental health field and psychiatry itself. After describing some ethnospecific services – these are services aimed at specific ethnic groups – in mental health, I devote a section to surveying the problems faced by these services. Finally, I look at some aspects of the nature of the black response (as I see it) to racism in mental health. Throughout this chapter I keep looking back at the pattern of the struggle against racism during the course of the past twenty years or so in order to set the scene for the second and third parts of this book.

Part 2 '*Underlying themes*' starts with a long chapter – Chapter 3 (*Psychiatry and mental health from a transcultural perspective*). I begin by surveying the history of psychiatry (as the medicalisation of madness and distress), highlighting the influence of racism in this process. There are sub-sections on the construction of 'schizophrenia' and 'depression' as illnesses in western Europe which indicate the problems that arise when they are applied across cultural boundaries. Then I consider some aspects of the modern practice of psychiatry, and go on to explore the meaning of 'spirituality' in relation to mental health, calling on 'Buddhist spirituality' as a concept that helps – at least has helped me – in understanding what is meant by this term in this day and age. That discussion leads naturally on to a section that I call 'holistic thinking' – a term designed to highlight some of the issues that point to practical problems in applying western psychiatry in a multicultural setting – and to a section about beliefs.

The sixth section of Chapter 3 covers the topic of psychotherapy and counselling seen from a transcultural perspective that takes on board issues of racism. And in the last section of this chapter I present a brief account of how I see mental health being represented in two systems of medicine that are much older and more popular (in terms of the numbers of people who access them) even now than western medicine (including psychiatry); these are Ayurveda and Chinese traditional medicine. Admittedly both these systems have been underdeveloped and even actively suppressed during the past one hundred years as a result of western domination and consequent 'westernisation' of the world. However, I believe that their study is warranted to gain some understanding of mental health and ways of dealing with mental health problems in a multicultural setting, such as those in modern western societies.

The aim of Chapter 4 (*Psychiatric stigma and racism*) is not to add to the already massive literature on stigma, but to examine the concept of psychiatric stigma in relation to the manifestations of racism in the mental health field, particularly the practice of psychiatry. By doing this, I hope to explore and understand why racism in psychiatry seems to persist so stubbornly in order to work out (in later chapters) how the struggle against it can be formulated. Since schizophrenia *par excellence* is the diagnosis that is stigmatised, I focus on this diagnosis.

Part 3 '*Changing practice*', contains two chapters. In Chapter 5 (*Moving forward*), I aim to see where and how movement is possible – hopefully by evolution rather than revolution, without too much upheaval. This chapter is largely about strategies for bringing about changes in psychiatry, in counselling and psychotherapy, in access to services and in psychiatric research. The four areas hang together and cannot be changed in isolation from each other. Also, I consider ways in which the voluntary sector may change for the better and directions for changes in research. In Chapter 6 (*Future prospects*), I try to take an optimistic view of the future without being too idealistic – keeping my feet on the ground. Here, I dare to present some ideas for the meaning of a multicultural mental health service, for a psychiatric service (within this model) that is sufficiently flexible to help people with mental health problems, for a model for psychotherapy and counselling that can be helpful to anyone who needs it, and for ways in which research may be structured so that it avoids the pitfalls inherent in a multicultural society in which racism is prevalent.

Part 1

Background

Chapter 1

Racism and cultural diversity

Racism exists in many societies in many different guises: as anti-Semitism in Europe, in the caste systems in India, within some aspects of Zionism in Palestine, etc. Even the conflict between people identified as 'Catholic' and 'Protestant' communities in Ireland is essentially based on the perception of people in racial terms as 'born' Catholics or Protestants. What Barzun (1965) calls 'race-thinking' appears to underpin many different conflicts today that are designated as 'ethnic conflicts'. But racism based on skin colour is the type of racism that predominates today in western Europe and North America.

The word 'culture', traditionally applied to an individual, usually refers to a mixture of behaviour and cognition arising from 'shared patterns of belief, feeling and adaptation that people carry in their minds' (Leighton and Hughes 1961: 447). The allusion to family culture or the culture of whole communities extends the meaning of the word further. Therefore, referring to a multiplicity of cultures (say in a multicultural society) implies cultural differences between groups of people – communities with different backgrounds, traditions and world views. Over recent years there has been an outpouring of literature on the topic of 'culture' and cultural studies (see bhabha 1994; Said 1994; Eagleton 2000). The understanding of the term 'culture' has changed. Culture is no longer seen as a closed system that can be defined very clearly, nor something that is composed of traditional beliefs and practices that are passed on from generation to generation, but as something living, dynamic and changing – a flexible system of values and world views that people live by and create and re-create continuously. It is a system by which people define their identities and negotiate their lives. So, understanding culture, training in cultural understanding or learning about cultures other than one's own, is about seeking an awareness of group norms collectively being created in the here-and-now in a context of the here-and-now.

Since 'ethnicity' is a popular concept for discussions about the multicultural and multi-racial nature of society, some comments on the term may be helpful. 'The term ethnicity acknowledges the place of history, language and culture in the construction of subjectivity and identity, as well as the fact that all discourse is placed, positioned, situated, and all knowledge is contextual' (Hall 1992: 257). In practical shorthand, the term 'ethnic' is taken to mean (at least in Britain) a mixture of cultural background and racial designation, the significance of each being variable. (It was, and still is, used differently on mainland Europe.) It is essentially about self-perception – how people see themselves – that takes on board the diversity of subjective positions, experience and histories of people. From a sociological point of view (e.g. Hall 1992; Malik 1996; Cohen 1999), the contemporary situation in Britain is seen as a shift into the construction of 'new ethnic identities' (Hall 1992: 256), new *British* ethnicities composed of people who see themselves (and are perceived) as adhering to ethnic groups that are different to the majority 'white' population. Stuart Hall (1992) sees this shift as a 'change from a struggle over the relations of representation to a politics of representation itself' (1992: 253). While at one time the term 'black was coined as a way of referencing the common experience of racism and marginalisation in Britain', today ethnicity is 'predicated on difference and diversity' (1992: 258). It should be noted that some writers have objected to this shift as deflecting attention away from 'broad structural processes including racism' in discussions about problems in health research and service provision (Stubbs 1993: 40). The point that needs grasping is that the importance of racism has not diminished. But instead of being a unitary concept that *per se* defines all problems, the central issue of race is 'constantly crossed and recrossed by the categories of class, of gender and ethnicity' (Hall 1992: 255).

This chapter considers very briefly the history of a black presence in the UK and other European countries. Then, it discusses the nature of racism, mainly in relation to the UK but touching on the European scene in general. The issues around multiculturalism, again mainly in relation to the British situation, will lead on to a consideration of ethnic issues in the mental health

field. These refer mainly to black people being excessively diagnosed as 'schizophrenic', over-represented among people who are
'sectioned' (involuntarily committed to hospital) and apprehended
in excessive numbers by the police as 'mentally ill', not referred for
psychotherapy, and so on. All these issues have been known for
over twenty years and commented upon extensively (see Fernando
2002), and so they are not described here in detail. A significant
development in the 1980s and 1990s was the arrival on the mental
health scene of services that aimed to provide specific services for
black and other minority ethnic groups – 'ethnic-specific services'. I
make some comments about these services, describing a few in
some detail. Finally, I discuss issues around race and culture in
psychiatric research and end by making some general conclusions.

Ethnic minorities in Europe

There are isolated reports of black people in Britain during Roman
times (Fryer 1984) but black communities as such were not evident
in Britain until about the mid-eighteenth century. Initially, these
communities were formed of African slaves brought back from the
West Indies as servants, later joined by Asian servants brought
back from India by returning nabobs – white people from Britain
who made fortunes in India (Baron 2001). Later, African and
Asian seamen employed in British ships settled in various ports.
Thus, the most long-standing British communities identifiable
today as 'black' or 'Asian' are descendents of African and Asian
seamen who settled locally, traders, and escaped or freed slaves;
they are located in or near formerly active seaports such as London
and Liverpool in England, and Cardiff in Wales. However, the
descendants of black Caribbean, African and Asian migrants of the
1950s and 1960s and their families now form most of Britain's
settled black communities. As a result of increasingly stringent
controls on immigration into Britain applied from the mid-1970s
onwards, recent arrivals who may be included within the designation of 'black' or 'Asian' are nearly all refugees (or people seeking
asylum) and families of British residents who are allowed in usually
after intensive vetting to establish that they are not 'economic
migrants'. On the whole, settled black and Asian British communities have spread from their original areas of settlement in
cities to the suburbs and, in the case of middle-class and business
people, to rural areas of Britain. Although refugees and asylum

seekers have tended to settle in London, a policy of dispersal was instituted in 2000 to send new arrivals to various parts of the UK (Home Office 1998), a policy that led to serious suffering (Audit Commission 2000). Thus, sizeable black communities are now present in several cities including, for example, Glasgow, Leeds and Newcastle.

It is difficult to estimate the numbers of black people in Europe since most European countries do not collect figures on the ethnic breakdown of their populations. The European Union (EU) comprises fifteen countries at the time of writing, in 2002. Melotti (1997) calculates that 11.5 million residents of these countries are immigrants from outside the EU, 90 per cent of them (about 10.3 million) coming from industrially underdeveloped countries. Germany, France and the UK, in that order, rank highest for these non-European immigrants. However, these figures do not address the fact that a large number of black and Asian people living in the EU today are citizens of the countries in which they reside. In 1995, as part of my involvement in an informal group of workers in the mental health field (called 'The Platform on Mental Health'), I collected information on ethnic minorities through contacts in various European locations. The figures (which have not been previously published) indicated that the number of 'black Europeans' numbered over 12 million in 1995 (Table 1.1). The numbers have obviously gone up since then and so today there are more black Europeans than there are white Swedes or Belgians.

The extent to which black Europeans are socially excluded and suffer from other forms of discrimination must vary from place to place. The Institute of Race Relations Race Audit Project, Statewatch (website: http://www.statewatch.org), that documents overt racism based on press cuttings and other information, is seldom short of reports of racial attacks on black people in nearly all European countries. Its January 2002 issue reports that racist and anti-Semitic violence in France 'is on the increase, reaching its highest level since 1990' (Institute of Race Relations 2002a: 7). School children seem particularly at risk of being attacked in Brandenburg in Germany (Institute of Race Relations 2002b: 11). Notwithstanding these (and other) signs of overt racism, it should be noted that all European countries, like Britain, have traditions of liberalism and resistance against persecution of people on racial grounds, and the EU has set its face against overt personal racism, for example by proposing that the lowest maximum penalty for

Table 1.1 Ethnic minorities, including refugees and asylum seekers, in
some European countries, approximate figures in 1995

	Percentage in total population (number in millions)	
	Settled ethnic minorities	All ethnic minorities
The Netherlands	7.6 (1.2)	8.1 (1.8)
UK	4.7 (2.7)	5.5 (3.2)
Denmark	1.6 (0.1)	3.1 (0.2)
Germany	4.0 (3.2)	4.6 (3.7)
France	5.4 (3.1)	6.2 (3.6)
Total	4.7 (10.3)	5.7 (12.5)

incitement to racial violence or hatred should be two years
imprisonment in all EU countries (European Union Institutions
2001), although it has so far taken no action on institutional
racism.

Nature of racism

The era of colonialism and the Atlantic slave trade was the time
when long-standing prejudices based on concepts of 'race' –
especially skin-colour race – became integrated as racism into
Euro-American culture, including the culture of psychiatry and
psychology (Fernando 1988). In his analysis of the connection
between racism and colonialism, Frantz Fanon (1967) has shown
very clearly how 'vulgar racism in its biological form' (1967: 35),
corresponding to a period of crude exploitation, changed into
'cultural racism' – 'a more sophisticated form [of racism] in which
the object is no longer the physiology of the individual but the
cultural style of a people' (McCulloch 1983: 120). This cultural
racism, deeply embedded in European culture, is represented in
western social and political systems as institutional racism of
modern times. Today institutional racism and racial prejudice at a
personal level exist together interacting with each other and
affecting society in many different ways. However, since various
meanings have been attributed over the years to the phenomenon
of racism there is now a 'crisis of meaning' for the concept. As Omi
and Winant (1994) state 'Today, the absence of a clear "common
sense" understanding of what racism means has become a significant obstacle to efforts aimed at challenging it' (1994: 70).

Innumerable theories of racism have been put forward and descriptions of its effects abound. In his book, *Racist Culture*, Goldberg (1993) argues against treating racism as a homogenous phenomenon:

> It follows that there may be different racisms in the same place at different times; or different racisms in various different places at the same time; or, again, different racist expressions – different that is, in the conditions of their expression, their forms of expression, the objects of their expression, and their effects – among different people at the same space-time conjuncture.
>
> (1993: 91)

Thus, racism during American slavery differs from post-slavery segregationism and each from current expressions of racism in the United States (US). Racism in South Africa during the times of apartheid differs from that expressed through inherent economic inequalities in the post-apartheid era. Nineteenth-century British racism in the colonies differs from current manifestations of racism in the UK. Yet some generalisation of the concept (of racism) is possible – hence the justification for its use: 'Concepts that are articulated resonate beyond the sites in which they were created' (Goldberg and Essed 2002: 3). Racism does not just exist as an abstract concept; its importance lies in its relevance to social relations between people. While racism cannot be adequately explained in abstraction from social relations nor can it be explained by reducing it to social relations (Hall 1980).

Essed (1990) has developed the concept of 'everyday racism' that is very much about the personal experience of racism in the course of day-to-day interactions between people. The people who exhibit racism are not necessarily overtly (racially) prejudiced, although if one examined their attitudes in some depth racist attitudes may be uncovered. Their unwitting racism may be implemented through ways of behaving and socialising. But if this approach is taken further, racism may be manifested in social and political systems because people unwittingly collude in it, possibly they gain from doing so. Wellman (1977) argues in *Portraits of White Racism*, that once racial prejudice is embedded within the structures of society, individual prejudice is no longer the problem, 'prejudiced people are not the only racists' (1977: 1). The idea of 'institutional racism' first appeared in a book by Carmichael and Hamilton (1997), *Black Power. The Politics of Liberation in America*. An inquiry into police failure in London to investigate the murder of a black teenager (Home Department 1999) defines institutional racism in terms of its practical effects – the 'collective failure of an organisation to provide an appropriate and professional service' (1999: 28). The problem, however, with this concept is that it seems to exclude the personal impact of racism on the individual and may *appear* to take responsibility for it away from the individual. However, recognising the main problem of racism as 'institutional' does not abrogate personal responsibility for racism. Anyone involved in a system that is institutionally racist is accountable, liable and blameable for their actions with special responsibility falling on those at the top of any system that is racist.

Modern racism

The lack of precision in defining racism results in much argument about its nature in the world of today – to the extent of questioning its very existence as a problem. Recently, when asked about the fact that only two of the eleven players chosen for its (cricket) test team were black – although 98 per cent of the population were black – the vice-chairman of Zimbabwe Cricket Union, while agreeing that black participation in the game was poor, said 'I don't like the word racism. It's unfair. I wish it would go away' (Meldrum 2001). Omi and Winant (1994) argue that a part of the problem arises from racism being seen as either an ideological phenomenon (with beliefs, attitudes, doctrines and discourse) that result in unequal and unjust practices, or as a structural phenomenon (with economic stratification, residential segregation, and institutional forms of inequality) that then gives rise to ideologies of privilege. They argue that 'ideological beliefs have structural consequences and social structures give rise to beliefs', so that racial ideology and (racist) social structure 'mutually shape the nature of racism in a complex, dialectical and overdetermined manner' (1994: 74–5). In fact, an inextricable linkage existed even in the development of the overtly racist plantation slavery of the US – the linkages between racism on the one hand, and on the other, shortage of cheap labour, the elaboration of juridical and property rights, and attitudes of racial superiority (Hall 1980).

Thus, ideological racism gets articulated through changing structural forms, and structural racism gets connected with changing ideologies. In such an open, flexible system, manifestations and locations of racism change constantly, especially in the face of opposition. Racism that was once openly applied in racial language is now applied in cultural language or the language of religion. Thus, instead of stating – or implying – that 'other races' are inferior, possess some unsavoury characteristic or pose a threat to social cohesion, the reference is to 'other' cultures, religions, ethnic groups or kinds of people, thought of in the same way as 'races', that is of groups that are unchanging and easily recognisable usually by physical appearance. Racism against Jews, namely anti-Semitism, is in fact hostility towards (what is perceived as) a racial group although defined in terms of religion; religious practice and belief do not come into it. In recent times 'alien cultures' have been seen as a danger to British society, for example by Margaret Thatcher in 1978 when she talked of Britain being 'swamped by people with a different culture' (Fitzpatrick 1990: 249). And even more recently, especially since the attack on New York in September 2001, Islam (a religion) is being used in similar racial idiom, with victimisation being justified on the grounds of preventing 'terrorism'.

One could visualise racism as an influence that permeates through a system hitching on to anything suitable for its purposes – any ideology, any discrimination, any facet of social functioning, any system of care, any educational enterprise, any construction of knowledge, etc. Racism then gets expressed through ideas of liberalism or democracy, culture or religion, conservatism or totalitarianism, gender differentiation, health care, psychological theories, medical systems, etc. So, in British society, racism – or perhaps racisms – takes, or take, diverse forms. The 'everyday racism' described by Essed (1990) merges into racial harassment and racial attacks which are still rife in many parts of the UK and on the European continent. Readers should see Virdee (1997) for a general survey, Collins (2001) on harassment of health service staff, Commission for Racial Equality (1987) for analysis of racial attacks in the UK, Carf (1997) for the death toll from racism in Europe, and Bjorgo (1997) for a survey of racism in Scandinavia. Although it is true to say that overt racial discrimination at a personal level – street racism – has declined over the past ten years in Britain (although this may not be the case in other European countries) it is still experienced in varying degrees by many black people in their everyday interactions with others. But it is the racism implemented through British institutional processes – institutional racism – that is proving most difficult to address.

Racism in the National Health Service was documented as long ago as 1983 (Commission for Racial Equality 1983) and studied in some depth (Anwar and Ali 1987). At that time, racism was approached mainly as personal prejudice but a recent book edited by Naz Coker (2001) points to the entrenched nature of institutional racism in the field of medicine. In this publication, Aneez Esmail (2001) points out how difficult it has been to research issues of racial discrimination in the admission of students to medical schools – not least because of political pressures aimed at preventing information on research getting into the public domain; Paramjit Gill (2001) describes the problems faced by black and Asian general practitioners because of racism; and Lyndsey Unwin (2001) outlines the complex ways in which institutional racism affects career progression in the National Health Service. A survey by the Association of University Teachers, quoted in a newspaper article (Major 2002), found that a third of ethnic minority university staff 'reported that they had experienced harassment on ethnic or racial grounds', and significantly points to serious 'racial discrepancies in the pay and conditions of staff' (2002: 9).

Racism and health services

Ahmad (1993) has shown how racism has manifested itself in the British health field through prominent health campaigns such as the 'Stop Rickets Campaign' and the 'Asian Mother and Baby Campaign', and also in less well-known campaigns such as the one against the use of surma (an eye cosmetic). In the case of rickets, when this condition emerged in the 1970s as prevalent among Asian children, it was seen as an Asian disease – 'Asian rickets'. When it was prevalent among white children, rickets had been counteracted through various simple means, such as fortifying margarine with vitamin D, but the remedy for Asian rickets was an educational and 'cultural' one: for example, an article in the *Lancet* (Goel *et al.* 1981) proposed 'health education' and a change towards the western diet and lifestyle. This happened because, once identified as being of Asian origin, Asian habits and genetics were blamed for its incidence – it was seen as a disease 'explained in terms of un-British eating and living habits, and perhaps a genetic deficiency in absorbing vitamin D into the bloodstream or in synthesizing vitamin D from sunlight' (Ahmad 1993: 21). When causes are identified as being located within 'culture', solutions are also 'cultural' – with 'culture' being seen (incorrectly) as an immutable fixed property of a group of people – in fact confounding 'culture' with 'race'.

Various books (Thomas and Sillen 1972; Richards 1997; Fernando 1988, 2002; Howitt and Owusu-Bempah 1994) have traced the diverse manifestations of racism in psychiatry and psychology – often masquerading as 'genetic' or 'cultural' observations or deductions. In the nineteenth and twentieth centuries black slaves in the American south, who absconded from bondage, were diagnosed as suffering from a disease causing them to run away, which was called 'drapetomania' (Cartwright 1851). A classic text on adolescence by a renowned American psychologist, Stanley Hall, included a chapter on 'Adolescent Races' in which Indians, Africans and North American 'Aborigines' were likened to immature children who 'live a life of feeling, emotion and impulse' (Hall 1904: 80). Kraepelin, the so-called 'father of modern psychiatry' (Weber and Engstrom 1997: 1), thought that depression was rare among Javanese people because they were immature (Kraepelin 1921). After a visit to the US, Carl Jung (1930), the eminent Swiss psychologist, postulated a theory that '[white] Americans descending from European stock have arrived at their striking peculiarities' as a result of 'racial infection' contracted by living in close proximity to black people (1930: 195). A renowned British colonial psychiatrist, J. C. Carothers (1953), writing in a monograph for the World Health Organisation, described (what he saw as) the African's 'lack of personal integration' (1953: 106), attributed the alleged rarity of depression among Africans to their lack of 'a sense of responsibility' (1953: 148) and postulated 'frontal [lobe] idleness' among Africans (1953: 161) as an underlying psychological deficiency. Also, an eminent psychiatrist and researcher, Leff (1973), hypothesised a theory of emotional differentiation which stated that '[people from] developed countries show a greater differentiation of emotional states than [do people from] developing countries' (1973: 305), except for African Americans who resemble the latter. In his book, Leff presented his theory as representing an evolutionary process (Leff 1981: 66).

Today, overt and obvious racism in the field of mental health is rare but institutional racism is widely prevalent. As in society at large, racism works through processes and procedures within systems and ways of thinking that underlie them. Institutional racism within psychiatry and psychology is a major problem in this respect. One source of institutional racism in psychiatry is the carry over of themes openly canvassed in the past, such as the image of black people being underdeveloped white people. The effect of thinking along these lines is evident in the persistence of the racist IQ movement within psychology and psychiatry, and the assumptions about emotional development in theories such as that propounded by Leff (1973) and discussed above. Another theme from the past that may partially explain the under-diagnosis of depression among black people (see later under 'Ethnic issues in mental health') is the psychiatric 'fact' (sic) repeatedly stated in the past that black people were unable to experience depression because, for example, they were 'irresponsible, unthinking, and easily aroused to happiness' (Green 1914: 703) or they lacked a 'sense of responsibility' (Carothers 1953: 148). In a modern context this theme appears in the 'finding' by Bebbington and colleagues (1981) that the incidence of depression among black people is lower than that among whites because they 'respond to adversity with cheery denial' (1981: 51). These themes are of course seldom expressed openly but nevertheless they determine diagnostic practice. I have found on numerous occasions that events, such as suicidal behaviour, or alleged 'lack of drive' are interpreted as bizarre behaviours indicative of schizophrenia in the case of black clients – something most unlikely in the case of white people.

A major problem in both clinical practice and research is that assumptions about black and Asian people and stereotypes about them, often coupled with misunderstandings, influence diagnostic practice. Some examples are the stereotypes of dangerousness (feeding into racist perceptions underlying the over-diagnosis of schizophrenia in black people); the view of Asian women as inherently passive because of their underdeveloped culture (promoting the failure to identify mental health problems in Asian women); and the perception of Asian and black family life as reflecting pathological over-inclusiveness and/or enmeshment (leading to inappropriate interventions). A report of an inquiry into the deaths of three black men in Broadmoor Hospital (Special Hospitals Services Authority 1993) drew attention to the pervasive influence within psychiatry of the stereotype 'big, black and dangerous'.

These topics are discussed further in Chapter 3 when categorisation and diagnosis in western psychiatry are considered. However, it is not just the field of diagnosis – mainly by psychiatrists and psychologists – that is affected by racism. Once someone enters the psychiatric system in the mental health services, perceptions of their racial designation is a major factor in most, if not in all, settings and institutions in Britain, especially (in my experience) those places that assume or claim that they work on a colour-blind basis.

Racism in Europe

Whatever the final structure of the EU, individual governments have been getting together for several years in order to 'harmonise' policies on immigration. One of the main (unstated) aims of this approach appears to be the limitation of the numbers of people from African and Asian countries who settle in Europe – the 'Fortress Europe' approach (Gordon 1989; Pieterse 1991) clearly underpinned by racism. The current drive towards a united Europe has raised various issues about the black presence in Europe. Pieterse (1991) has (citing McBridge 1988) pointed out how the image of 'European culture' – 'from Plato to Nato' – that is being promoted politically ignores Europe's 'contemporary multicultural realities' (Pieterse 1991: 3–4). Discussions tend to be about including identities of states (France, Germany, Britain, etc.) seen in terms of traditional, 'official', nineteenth-century imperial forms. Pieterse (1991) writes that, as 'Fortress Europe' in association with NATO extends its sights southwards, Europe's relationship with Africa, Asia and South America is acquiring new dimensions: 'These problems also reflect on migrants of non-European origin within Europe, so they also run *through* Europe. . . . How minorities of non-European origin are viewed is affected by how Europe views itself in relation to the continents [of Asia, Africa and South America]' (1991: 6, italics in the original). In 1997, an opinion poll was carried out in the fifteen member states of the EU involving 16,154 persons (European Commission 1997). The development of a multicultural society was welcomed by 75 per cent of the people polled (although what this actually meant may have been interpreted differently in different countries), and 70 per cent considered that discrimination at work should be forbidden. However, against these liberal attitudes were other seriously worrying answers to the poll: 20 per cent agreed with wholesale repatriation of immigrants from non-EU countries (equivalent to black people), and 39 per cent did not agree with either their assimilation or their integration. The report on the survey concluded that 'feelings of racism co-exist with strong belief in democratic system and respect' (1997: 5).

In analysing immigration policies in Europe, Melotti (1997) points to differences in approach between France, the UK and Germany. He believes that the French approach is that of 'ethno-centric assimilation', essentially assimilation to become 'good Frenchmen [and women]' (1997: 76). The British, he says, practice a pragmatic approach that results in 'uneven pluralism'; according to his analysis '[cultural] differences of immigrants are . . . taken for granted, and the main concern is to make sure that immigrants cause as little damage as possible to the "British way of life"', although it is implicitly made clear that control remains in the hands of the 'majority'. Melotti calls the German approach 'insti-tutionalisation of precariousness', meaning that 'immigrants fundamentally remain foreigners' (1997: 81). Melotti believes that all these approaches are deeply rooted in the different political cultures. I agree that the differences in approach towards black people are indeed best seen in a historic context, but history does not necessarily dictate the future. The following paragraph presents a personal view based mainly on discussions with black Europeans I have met at conferences on mainland Europe and the contents of an important issue of the journal *Race and Class* edited by Sivanandan (1991).

There are marked differences in attitudes to racism and cultural difference in some European countries compared to those in Britain, almost certainly resulting from the nature of their contact with black people in the past, the attitude to their own 'culture', history of black migration into those countries, and the recent history, especially that of the overt racism (including anti-Semitism) of the 1930s and 1940s. The idea of cultural diversity is frowned upon in France because of the high status attributed to being (culturally) French. The tendency in France is to deny that 'race' makes any difference so long as one is culturally 'French' – although racism is rife. This means that a discussion of racism is more difficult in France than it is in the UK, and promotion of multiculturalism is a non-starter in France. In the Netherlands, integration of immigrants is given high priority, cultural differences are acceptable – even desirable – within Dutch society, but any mention of racism in the host community is met with embarrassment. Racism tends to be sidestepped rather than denied. In Germany, the very idea of racism raises hackles or else a frightened silence, intimating an unwillingness to engage with this matter at all. There, an undercurrent of suppressed, potentially violent racism is almost palpable to an outsider like me. And it is quickly and fearfully confirmed by black Germans and the few white German psychiatrists who have dared to confront the problem. Since the main black minority group in Germany is Turkish-Muslim, racism is muddled with anti-Muslim sentiments.

Today in France the accent is on cultural conformity; if one is culturally 'French' one can be any colour – or so the theory goes. So when racial (racist) differentiation occurs, it tends to be denied or wrapped up in political euphemisms or clouded by allusions to cultural deviancy. Thus, north Africans may be discriminated against because they are politically suspect – and now more than ever because they may be nominally Muslim. Indeed the current cultural dilemma for black people in France is consistent with that described so vividly by Fanon (1952) in *Peau Noire, Masques Blancs* (*Black Skin, White Masks*). Germany has a tradition of recognising nationality by 'blood', a biological construction of German nationhood. It is no accident that the legal obstructions to immigrants gaining citizenship – or even resident status – are immense. Anyone applying for citizenship has to show knowledge of the German language, have economic security, show an inclination to orientate themselves towards German 'culture' and way of life, etc. (Räthzel 1991). But when descendents of people who had left Germany to settle in parts of Russia wanted to return after the war, they were accepted as 'ethnic Germans', although some did not even speak the German language. On one of my visits to Germany I met a German-born man whose parents came from Turkey. He had been unable to obtain German citizenship but was working as a teacher of German to 'ethnic Germans' who had 'returned' from Russia (and had full German citizenship)! In the Scandinavian countries racism appears to be implemented at arms length as it were. It is perceived as an alien concept and purely a stance taken by some people for economic and political reasons. So institutional racism is not recognised at all and the tendency is to 'culturalise' or 'democratise' racism. For example, Quraishy and O'Connor (1991) describe how 'the cultural threat from the Third

World' (1991: 115) is discussed in Denmark as a political problem and Larsson (1991) observes how Swedish racism is expressed 'not in terms of racism or immigration, but as a question of "local democracy", where "ordinary people" can have a say in an increasingly controversial issue' (1991: 109).

Multiculturalism, racism and ethnicity

Racism has always been a problem for black and Asian people in the UK. In the 1950s the presence of black and Asian people was euphemistically referred to as 'the colour problem'; as immigration from Asia and Africa, mainly from ex-colonies that had achieved independence, was highlighted in the popular media as a 'problem' a new euphemism arose in the 1970s – the 'immigration problem'. As immigration controls were established, racism was exhibited in adverse comments about – and indeed overt hostility towards – refugees and asylum seekers, subsumed under what is presented in the media as a 'refugee problem' or the 'asylum seeker problem'. And now in the early years of the new millennium, there appears to be a revival of racism as part and parcel of a 'war against terrorism'. Today, racism is articulated in a mixture of ways that feed into and compound each other – in overt hostility to refugees and asylum seekers; in hostility to Muslims, which often extends towards non-Muslim people with brown skins, i.e. 'people who look different' (Singh 2001); in discrimination in the job market (Modood 1997), highlighted in a report prepared by the Performance and Innovation Unit (2001) for the Prime Minister; in student selection (McManus 1998); etc. However, the main and perhaps most serious problem is institutional racism that pervades all major systems affecting British people, including mental health services and the main disciplines that inform such services, namely psychology and psychiatry.

Yet, in parallel with continuing racism there has been a shift in Britain towards an acceptance of cultural plurality. In a British context cultural plurality, or multiculturalism, means that society is composed of many 'cultures', which in turn means that there are in society a multiplicity and variety of ways of life, world views, habits, ideologies, marriage customs, methods of child rearing, etc., all that goes to make up 'culture'. Many people in Britain seem comfortable with this plurality, accepting it as the norm for Britain, but there is sometimes a problem when it comes to verbalising this acceptance. I believe this happens because there is confusion as to the meaning of multiculturalism. When 'culture' is talked about, it is far too often perceived as something fixed and immutable – very much in the way 'race' is conceptualised. In discussions on the topic there is frequent slippage between words representing 'race' and those referring to 'culture'. The use of the term 'ethnic' often adds to the confusion. And when cultural groups are imagined as living side by side, interacting with one another but developing their own individual, separate cultures, multiculturalism is imagined as socially divisive. (For a detailed discussion of the terms race, culture and ethnicity, see Fernando 2002.) However, the reality today is that cultures are not clearly distinct from one another and 'cultural groups' do not live separate lives. Perhaps that has never been the case.

As black and Asian people became relatively numerous in Britain after the break-up of the British empire, the ways in which cultural groups related to one another mimicked the patterns established in the empire – the empire coming home. So, early on in the 1950s and 1960s, although social interaction across cultural divides was fostered, close associations between members of different cultural groups were not encouraged. Culturally 'mixed' marriages were frowned upon and children with such 'mixed' parentage faced discrimination from both sides, being referred to as 'mixed race', 'hybrid' or 'half-caste' in the classic conflation of 'race' and 'culture'. This gradually changed in the 1970s. People tended to take sides, either welcoming culturally and/or racially mixed partnerships as a way of resolving the 'colour problem' or harking back to myths and fears engendered by 'miscegenation'. Concepts such as 'culture clash' were postulated to explain individual and social problems of individuals perceived as belonging to 'two cultures', thereby implying that mixtures were problematic, almost pathological. And racism was largely ignored as a social problem for the whole of society – just one for black people to worry about.

The reality now is very different to that in the 1970s. At a personal level, cultures have not remained clearly distinct and partnerships and marriages across lines identified as 'racial' and/or 'cultural' have gradually increased in frequency over the years. Culturally 'mixed' partnerships are no longer frowned upon by most people. An analysis of the 1991 census by Berrington (1996) finds that 16 per cent of black men and 13 per cent of black women were living with a white partner at the time of the census – such relationships being more common among younger people and those born in the UK than among older people and people born abroad. Less than six years later, a survey by the Policy Studies Institute (Berthoud and Beishon 1997) found that half of black British-born Caribbean men and a third of women had white partners; for Indians and Asian people from Africa ('African Asian' according to the Policy Studies Institute nomenclature) 19 per cent of British-born men and 10 per cent of women had white partners. Black and Asian people have developed complex ways of building up their identities reflecting both their backgrounds and their residence in a multi-racial and multicultural Britain. And racism is recognised as a serious problem for British society as a whole, especially since the publication of the Macpherson Report in 1999 (Home Department 1999), which is discussed in Chapter 2.

So, cultural plurality (multiculturalism) means that British society draws on a variety – a diversity – of cultural roots and traditions, eastern and western, Asian, Caribbean, African, Chinese, Somali, etc. But, together with this sharing, there are still discernible minority 'cultural' groups or 'ethnic' groups that are becoming integrated into a plural society. In the field of health research and service provision it is useful and possible for practical purposes – for example in providing interpreter services, in identifying discriminatory processes or institutional racism, or in monitoring the use of compulsory powers within the mental health system – to categorise people into cultural groups (where culture alone is the criterion), racial groups (where traditional ideas of 'race', usually based on physical appearance, are used) or, most importantly, ethnic groups (where both 'race' and 'culture' are addressed in terms of its commonsense meaning linked to personal identity). Thus, the concept of ethnicity straddles both culture and race while the struggle against racism and the promotion of multiculturalism are two sides of the same coin (Figure 1.1).

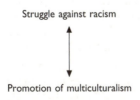

Struggle against racism

Promotion of multiculturalism

Figure 1.1 Racism and multiculturalism

Racial and cultural identity

The relationship between (what is understood as) 'race' and (what is understood as) 'culture' is changing in the real world – the world as experienced by ordinary people. For example, results of the Policy Studies Institute survey quoted earlier show that the proportion of 'black' children with both black and white parents is rising rapidly in the UK (Berthoud and Beishon 1997) and so there are increasing numbers of 'white' people with black ancestry and 'black' people with white ancestry. One's 'race' no longer indicates 'culture' with any accuracy at all and this leaves an opening for the increasing use of 'ethnicity' as a concept for categorisation and a locus for identity. Furthermore, there are other changes in ethnic consciousness in British society apart from those changes that evolved from 'race' and 'culture'; a growing consciousness of being a nationality within the UK is resulting in both black and white people identifying as Scottish, Welsh, Irish and English. These changes are reflected in the terminology used to locate identity – whether as individuals or as communities. In the 1950s and 1960s many immigrants from Asia, Africa and the Caribbean, and their children, were happy to identify as 'black people', although the more generic term 'ethnic minorities' was even then becoming popular to include black people as well as other minority 'immigrant' groups. In the 1980s and 1990s, additional identities were pursued denoting religious categories (e.g. Muslim or Sikh) but these were seldom perceived as alternatives to 'black' or 'Asian'. The result is that the term now generally used to describe what were 'black people' is 'black-and-Asian' with subdivisions reflecting geographical origins of both 'black' and 'Asian' into (say) 'Chinese', 'African', 'African-Caribbean', etc., or subdivisions reflecting religious affiliations of 'Muslim', 'Hindu', 'Sikh', etc. Ethnic groups have come to be seen as being within either the majority (white) category or the minority (black and Asian) category. Further (mainly) white people of Irish descent have begun to refer to their ethnicity as an important source of pride and sometimes discrimination by other white people. Some people with parents who are from different 'ethnic' groups are beginning to ask for recognition as being different to either. Indeed, the situation remains fluid and likely to change in response to events, particularly events that affect the manifestations of racism.

The concepts of culture, race and ethnicity have always been far from clear-cut. Therefore, the importance to people of how they feel with respect to these concepts – as cultural beings, racial beings or ethnic beings – reflects matters of deep significance. The situation in the late 1990s (compared to that in the 1970s) is that many black and Asian people – perhaps the majority of people who form the minority ethnic communities – think that (at a personal level) 'culture' matters more than 'race'. But, ever so often – far too often – continuing racism repeatedly reminds black and Asian people (whether seen as such by them or by others in society) that – as Cornel West (1994) states about the US – *Race Matters*, the colour of one's skin matters, how one is seen in racial terms matters. Thus, at a very personal level, the meaning of living in a multicultural society is repeatedly being interrupted by events and experiences that raise the issue of racism. Another dimension that is often ignored is that of social class. Sociologist Phil Cohen (1999) points to a split between people on the street (as it were) grappling with realities of discrimination in employment and housing and legal systems, and so-called 'culture-workers' (who include many professionals and writers); the latter 'view issues of race through a cultural lens' (1999: 8) in contrast to the former who think predominantly in racial terms. In this respect (as Cohen points out) The Stephen Lawrence Inquiry (Home Department 1999) was of particular significance because it brought together various dimensions of racism: street racism and cultural racism; overt racism and covert racism; direct racism and indirect racism; individual racism and institutional racism. In short the pursuit of multiculturalism always involves a struggle against racism.

Ethnic issues in mental health

Evidence of disadvantages suffered by black and Asian people in the mental health services became evident in the late 1970s and 1980s (see Fernando 1988; Mental Health Act Commission 1989, 1991; Webb-Johnson 1991). The inequalities identified since then are summarised in Box 1.1, based on a table in the book *Race and Culture in Psychiatry* (Fernando 1988) which was published about fifteen years ago. Since then, similar tables have been quoted elsewhere including a discussion document produced by the Home Office and Department of Health for the Reed Report on Secure Services (Department of Health and Home Office 1994). Also relevant statistics for London have been summarised by Bhui (2002). Each of the points listed depicted in Box 1.1 may well

Box 1.1 Ethnic issues in mental health services

Black and ethnic minorities are more often

1. diagnosed as schizophrenic
2. compulsorily detained under the Mental Health Act
3. admitted as 'offender patients'
4. held by police under Section 136 of the Mental Health Act
5. transferred to locked wards from open wards
6. not referred for psychotherapy
7. given high doses of medication
8. sent to psychiatrists by courts
9. have unmet needs

---

reflect complex issues of not just race and culture but also class, gender, poverty, etc., and so could be studied in depth – that is if only there are reliable data and objective measures that would render such study worthwhile. Also, the items may be analysed by looking at similarities and differences in statistics on diagnostic rates, for example, between those from the US, the UK and countries on mainland Europe, except that the nature of the items, such as diagnosis, are such that comparisons are likely to yield more questions than answers.

There is little doubt in my mind that the ethnic issues that have been highlighted arise from combinations of factors. First and foremost there is the fundamental issue of the validity of traditional psychiatric diagnoses. Since these are based on an ethnocentric western psychiatry their meaning transculturally is very uncertain; in fact their validity in any situation is questionable – a matter which is discussed later under the subheading 'Psychiatric research'. Then there is the matter of how the diagnoses are made both in clinical practice and in research studies. Psychiatry is not an objective science. A psychiatric assessment whereby symptoms are identified involves subjective judgements based on human values of the person making the diagnosis which in turn reflect their cultural background and mindset. This in itself may not be a great drawback if the judgements are consistent and applied without bias. But that is not the case. As Dickenson and Fulford (2000) observe 'in the areas of experience and behaviour with which psychiatry is concerned *human values are highly diverse*' (2002: 4, italics in original). In other words, these values are not easy to define and extremely variable.

What happens in psychiatry is that symptoms are identified and lead on to the delineation of 'phenomena'. The empirical approach whereby psychiatrists identify mental 'phenomena' that constitute 'psychopathology' (such as 'guilt', 'self-depreciation', 'depression', feelings of passivity', etc.) implies that they get through to a reality that is not just appearance; but these 'facts' (i.e. the presence or absence of psychopathology) are made under the influence of a socially constructed reality and culture (Harari 2001), and reflect the world views and values of the psychiatrist together with the assumptions that underpin the 'culture' of psychiatry itself (see Fernando 2002). Thus, using a value-laden psychiatry derived in a relatively narrow cultural tradition is asking for trouble. When racism comes into the picture the trouble becomes potentially dangerous. So, it is unlikely that there is a simple answer to these 'ethnic issues' or that one or two research projects can unravel them. The best that can be said at present is that a greater under-standing of what culture and cultural diversity mean in the application of psychology and psychiatry may enable practitioners and researchers to understand what may be going on; and that evaluating the ways in which racism in all its forms affects both disciplines – and indeed the systems that deliver mental health care – can bring them nearer to lessening the inequities that are currently seen as 'ethnic issues'. In other words, ethnic issues represent a complex mixture of 'cultural' and 'racial' issues that require exploration and understanding.

I do not intend to even try to develop a comprehensive theory to explain these ethnic issues. Suffice it to note for the purposes of this chapter that (a) overall, the issues depicted in Box 1.1 are as real in 2002 as they were in 1988; (b) it is the totality of the items taken together that speaks strongly, pointing to the importance of racism and failure to address cultural diversity in mental health services; and (c) since mental health services are underpinned by the disciplines of psychiatry and psychology, it is these fields of practice and knowledge that require examination and reform primarily. The issues are sometimes complex but on the whole similar to those underlying other race issues – for example the over-representation of black people in prison and the excessive exclusion from school of black children.

One of the central issues for the diagnostic system that psychiatry currently uses is the relatively high rate at which 'schizophrenia' is diagnosed among black people in the UK. I believe that this issue lies at the centre of the problems in the mental health services that present as ethnic issues. If we can unravel this central problem, some of the issues about 'cultural insensitivity' may fall away and we may be able to move forward in a way that will bring results that are lasting. Another issue that carries considerable practical importance, but which is more at the 'soft' end of the mental health services, is that of psychotherapy and counselling. As indicated in Box 1.1, relatively few black people seem to be referred for psychotherapy or counselling but, even more importantly, when they are referred there is considerable dissatisfaction with the approaches in the 'therapies' they receive. Therefore, instead of describing and analysing all the issues given in Box 1.1, I merely and briefly review these two fields within mental health – the diagnosis of schizophrenia and psychotherapy/counselling.

Schizophrenia

Reports of a relatively high rate of black in-patients being diagnosed as 'psychotic' appeared in the US during the latter part of the nineteenth century (e.g. Babcock 1895). Pasamanick (1963), noting that non-white rates for 'psychosis' were higher than those for whites in state hospitals, observed that, between 1920 and 1955, there was a change in the style of diagnosis of black people in the US: the diagnosis of schizophrenia increased while that of manic depression (bipolar disorder) decreased. Similar findings were reported in the US in 1950s and 1960s (e.g. Wilson and Lantz 1957: Jaco 1960; Simon 1965). It seems well established that African-American patients (compared to their non-African-American counterparts) are more likely to be diagnosed as schizophrenic and less likely to be diagnosed as suffering from affective disorder (mania or depression) in various settings in the US (Strakowski *et al.* 1993; Strakowski *et al.* 1995; Mukherjee *et al.* 1983; Neighbors *et al.* 1989; Flaskerud and Hu 1992), although some doubt has been thrown on this by data from the Epidemiologic Catchment Area study in the US which reveals no significant differences in the rate at which schizophrenia is diagnosed between black and white patients, once the data were corrected for age, sex, socio-economic status and marital status (Adebimpe 1994). In reviewing the situation regarding race and mental disorder in the US, Adebimpe (1994) supports the contention that findings are 'confusing and inconclusive' (1994: 27), and suggests that black and white patients differ in their treatment experiences in various ways; these include treatment-seeking behaviour, likelihood of involuntary commitment, presentation of psychiatric symptoms and accuracy of psychological tests.

British studies in the 1960s and 1970s showed a disproportionately excessive number of black people being diagnosed as 'schizophrenic' (e.g. Bagley 1971; Cochrane 1977; Carpenter and Brockington 1980; Dean *et al*. 1981). A more recent survey of in-patients legally (compulsorily) detained in a hospital in Birmingham, UK, showed that about two-thirds of black, West Indian patients, as opposed to one-third of the whites, were diagnosed as 'schizophrenic' (McGovern and Cope 1987); and studies in Nottingham (Harrison *et al*. 1988; 1997) and London (King *et al*. 1994; Bhugra *et al*. 1997) confirmed that black people seen as patients in various settings were given the diagnosis of schizophrenia to a disproportionately excessive extent – twelve to thirteen times more often than expected in one study. The authors of the London and Nottingham studies argue that, by using the Present State Examination (Wing *et al*. 1974), commonly called the PSE, 'misdiagnosis' is avoided – the assumption being that the PSE masked any racist misconceptions that the diagnosticians may have held. Unfortunately, when racism is institutionalised in ways of working – as it undoubtedly is in the psychiatric system of making judgements about the presence or absence of 'symptoms' (see pp. 156–9) – use of the PSE cannot counter this because it does not incorporate any means of doing so.

Statistics on ethnic differences in the diagnosis of 'schizophrenia' in mainland Europe are sparse. My impression is that what happens in Britain is likely to be replicated elsewhere, and anecdotal reports I have received personally justify this impression. A disproportionately high diagnosis of schizophrenia has been reported among Surinamese immigrants living in The Netherlands (Selten *et al*. 1997) and among 'migrants' (foreign-born people) living in Germany (Haasen *et al*. 1996). In the case of Germany, 'immigrants' are likely to be predominantly of Turkish origin, who may not be immigrants at all but people who have been in the country for generations but unable to obtain German nationality.

The causes of, or the issues underlying, racially linked differences in rates of diagnosed 'illness' are probably complex and variable. An early study in New York attempting to elucidate the reasons for the excessive diagnosis of schizophrenia among black people in the US (Simon *et al*. 1973) concluded that 'the diagnostic differences found between blacks and whites were a reflection of US hospital psychiatrists' diagnostic habits [with regard to Blacks] as much as anything else' (1973: 511); and one in Britain (Littlewood and Lipsedge 1982) indicated that atypical syndromes among black patients may be 'misdiagnosed' as schizophrenia. Also, Bromberg and Simon (1968) in the US observed that (what they call) 'protest psychosis', essentially an expression of anger among black Americans by repudiating white people and their social structures, may be 'misdiagnosed' as 'schizophrenia'. Allon (1971) reported that, when a distinction is established in diagnosis between 'process schizophrenia' and 'reactive schizophrenia' (the former seen as having a relatively high 'genetic' component), black African Americans were disproportionately given the diagnosis of process schizophrenia – suggesting that stereotyping of black people as genetically inferior may play a part in diagnostic discrepancies. Over fifty years ago, St Clair (1951) noted difficulties encountered by white psychiatrists in the US in comprehending, and therefore evaluating properly, the feelings and behaviour of black people because of mutual mistrust and hostility between racial groups. All this pointed to issues around bias.

In the UK, Parkman and colleagues (1997) reported that black patients in south London expressed less satisfaction with mental health services than did white patients, and several reports now indicate that many African Americans, including mental hospital in-patients, are mistrustful of mental health service providers (Whaley 2001). Koffman and colleagues (1997), reviewing ethnic differences in use of beds in the mental health services, point to a potential for racial discriminatory practice in the psychiatric services in London. Strakowski and colleagues (1997), comparing clinical diagnoses made at an American emergency service with those made for research purposes, found that racially determined diagnostic inaccuracies (leading to inappropriate diagnosis of schizophrenia in black patients) may result because clinical psychiatrists do not elicit adequate information from black patients. After studying ways in which judgements about the presence or absence of specific symptoms are related to the final diagnosis, Trierweiler and colleagues (2000) concluded that clinicians attribute and weigh particular observations differently for patients of different races. According to that study, clinicians tend to attribute the presence of (what they consider to be) 'negative symptoms' and 'delusions' to 'schizophrenia' in the case of black patients more often than they do in the case of white patients. All this points to issues of misunderstanding and mistrust.

The issue of bias in diagnostic style is a difficult matter to research using traditional methodology, and it is difficult to get funding for studies using unconventional methods. A study by Loring and Powell (1988) is an exception in this respect. In a study using carefully constructed vignettes (of case histories) they researched the diagnostic approaches of 290 black and white American psychiatrists. They concluded that (a) overall, black clients, compared to white clients, were given a diagnosis of schizophrenia more frequently by both black and white clinicians – although this was done to a lesser extent by the former; and (b) all the clinicians appeared to ascribe violence, suspiciousness and dangerousness to black clients even though the case studies were the same as those for the white clients. An attempt to carry out a similar – but much less extensive – study in the UK (Lewis *et al.* 1990) was flawed (something obviously not picked up by peer review!) through the researchers' apparent lack of sophistication in handling the issue of 'race' (Fernando 1991). The researchers used just one vignette (varied four ways by altering the stated race and gender) and this carried within it elements that raised images of race (apart from stated designation of race), thereby invalidating the usefulness of the vignette.

In Britain black people in psychiatric hospitals are seen as 'dangerous' without adequate objective reasons (Harrison *et al.* 1984) and black patients are over-represented among compulsorily detained patients in hospital (Ineichen *et al.* 1984; McGovern and Cope 1987). In the US too, there is an over-representation of blacks as involuntary commitments to public mental institutes (Lindsey and Paul 1989; Lawson *et al.* 1994). The concluding remarks by Loring and Powell (1988) (whose study is quoted above) are worth repeating here. They point out that black and white people are 'seen differentially even if they exhibit the same behaviour', and that 'these differences will be reflected and legitimized in official statistics on psychopathology' (1988: 19). The lessons are clear: unless we look at institutional processes, we are unlikely to find out why and how diagnoses reflect and perpetuate racism.

Psychotherapy and counselling

Ethnic statistics on the use of psychotherapy and counselling services in the UK are non-existent, although anecdotal evidence shows that people from black and Asian communities are seldom referred for such therapy in the National Health Service (Campling 1989). A high drop-out rate from psychotherapy was reported many years ago in the case of black patients in the US (e.g. Rosenthal and Frank 1958; Yamamoto *et al.* 1967, 1968) and it is likely that a similar situation exists in Britain too. Yet research in this area is not straightforward. The question is not just about access to services providing psychotherapy and counselling but more importantly the nature of what is offered as 'psychotherapy' or 'counselling'. One needs to consider the appropriateness of the therapy in terms of models used in understanding (or helping the clients to understand) the problems presented, the attitudes and ideologies of the people who provide 'therapy', and so on. Outcome in the case of psychotherapy and counselling is even more difficult to measure than it is in the case of physical therapies and evaluating benefit is equally difficult.

Psychotherapy or counselling for people from black, Asian and other minority ethnic communities must be geared to their needs, must use models that are consistent with their cultural backgrounds, and should be carried out by people who are able to make constructively therapeutic relationships with clients from these communities. In this type of mental health service, more than in any other, the nature of the training undergone by the therapist and indeed many personal qualities of the therapist are both crucial aspects of the quality of the service itself. So, issues are not merely about access to psychotherapy services but are also about the appropriateness of what is offered as counselling or psychotherapy – and that means that the training of psychotherapists and counsellors must be in keeping with the multi-ethnic nature of society. There is little doubt that the scene, as far as black communities are concerned, is dire. The dissatisfaction with traditional psychiatry that dominates the statutory mental health services sometimes leads black people to suppose that 'talking therapies' are the answer. Yet anecdotal evidence suggests that many black people are disappointed with psychotherapy and counselling provided at generic centres, whether private, voluntary or statutory. However, I know from talking to people working at ethnic-specific counselling centres (i.e. those that aim to provide counselling for specific ethnic groups) in the 'black voluntary sector' and clients attending them that such centres often have a high degree of client satisfaction. Later in this book I discuss general aspects of some of these centres

('Initiatives in mental health service provision', Chapter 2), the problems they encounter ('Problems of the black voluntary sector', Chapter 2) and ways in which they function ('Psychotherapy and counselling', Chapter 3).

Psychiatric research

There are many fundamental problems with psychiatric research generally and I shall summarise them briefly. The first problem arises at the point of planning the questions to be asked. Psychiatric research, more than research in any other field of medicine, is politically driven. Today, the pharmaceutical companies tend to fund much psychiatric research, either directly or indirectly. Therefore, most research that is published tends to focus on the use of drugs rather than on any other form of therapy. Research into service provision is also problematic. As government policies emphasise safety of the public over the human rights of psychiatric patients, researching 'assertive outreach' achieves prominence over passive user-friendly community care. The second major problem is about the reliance on diagnosis as a basis for categorisation of subjects who are researched. In a multicultural society, few, if any, diagnostic categories currently used can claim scientific validity – and this lack of validity applies mostly to schizophrenia, the category most used. The third group of problems centres on methodology generally used in research. On the whole these are culture-blind and blind to the effects of racism. Even more importantly, methods tend to be blind to the serious drawbacks of relying on empiricism as a scientific foundation for research in psychiatry (Harari 2001). Most psychiatric research today starts off by marshalling so-called observable measurable data, assuming that all the data are value free – or at least reasonably 'objective'. However, this is far from the case. For example, when Sandor (2001) wrote in a paper in the *Psychiatric Bulletin* that 'home treatment' (treatment provided in a patient's home that is usually valued by users of services) lacks a 'strong evidence-based rationale' (2001: 486), a psychiatric registrar wrote in to point out that 'it is imperative that we embrace the challenge to measure what is important' (McCauley 2002: 155). Apart from simple items, such as age and gender, etc. measurable data that are then manipulated to provide wide-ranging conclusions are heavily value laden (see under 'Ethnic issues in mental health') and theory laden (see Harari 2001). Moreover, those items that are measured as 'phenomena' (such as depression, thought disorder and hallucination) are not objective 'facts' although they are often treated as such. Further, psychiatric data – unlike data in natural sciences – are similar to data in social psychology where they (the data) deal in events that fluctuate markedly over time, but are presented as 'facts' (Gergen 1973). For example, the propensity to aggressiveness, or feelings of depression, or 'hearing voices' may be noted as relatively stable 'observations' about a person and conclusions drawn about him or her, ignoring the reality that the events that were construed (as aggressiveness, feelings of depression, hallucinations) may well be context related and transitory.

It would be evident from the previous paragraph that when it comes to cross-cultural research, especially research that is presented as 'epidemiological' research (measuring incidence or prevalence of illnesses as defined within western psychiatry), the problems are immense. The main issue is around the question of validity of diagnoses – their usefulness when used across cultures. Kleinman (1977) has called this the problem of 'category fallacy' (1977: 4), and describes it with respect to the diagnosis of depression as follows.

> The depressive syndrome represents a small fraction of the entire field of depressive phenomena. It is a cultural category constructed by psychiatrists in the West to yield a homogeneous group of patients. By definition, it excludes most depressive phenomena even in the West because they fall outside its narrow boundaries. Applying such a category to analyse cross-cultural studies, or even in direct field research, is not a cross-cultural study of depression, because by definition it will find what is 'universal' and systematically miss what does not fit its tight parameters. The former is what is seen and therefore 'seen' by a Western cultural model; the latter, which is not so defined and therefore not 'seen', raises far more interesting questions for cross-cultural research.
>
> (1977: 3–4)

Kleinman's arguments apply even more cogently to diagnoses such as schizophrenia. The basic problem is that the psychiatric system having developed within a specific tradition – broadly termed 'western culture' (see Fernando 1995b) – the particular illness model (with its diagnoses) that is applied reflects the world view about the human condition within that tradition. The situation *vis-à-vis* a different cultural tradition may be very different. One could argue that if a system – the psychiatric system in this case – is sufficiently flexible it could take on changes in world view to suit each particular situation, but this is not the case. The basic syndromes agreed as 'illnesses' are adhered to as unchanging and, even more importantly, the main symptoms recognised are perceived as 'phenomena' that have an existence of their own. Kleinman suggests that an ideal cross-cultural study should begin with phenomenological descriptions that are indigenous to each cultural group. He believes that researchers may then 'elicit and compare symptom terms and illness labels independent of a unified framework' (1977: 4).

The International Pilot Study of Schizophrenia

The main problems of cross-cultural research can be illustrated by considering a well-known study conducted by the World Health Organisation, the International Pilot Study of Schizophrenia (World Health Organisation 1973, 1979), commonly called the IPSS. The diagnostic method used in this study was based on the PSE described by its founder, Wing (1978), as 'a special technique of interviewing patients, known as the Present State Examination (PSE), which is simply a standardized form of the psychiatric diagnostic interview ordinarily used in Western Europe, based on a detailed glossary of differential definitions of symptoms' (1978: 103). The PSE has been likened to a telescope (Wing 1985); 'within its specifications it can be used by trained people to look for a limited range of phenomena' (1985: 326). The IPSS assumed that the categorisation system developed within Europe (in a western cultural setting) was applicable universally, and set out to establish a reliable method of diagnosing schizophrenia (in western terms). Nine centres, namely Aarhus (Denmark), Agra (India), Cali (Colombia), Ibadan (Nigeria), London (UK), Moscow (USSR), Prague (Czechoslavakia), Taipeh (Taiwan) and Washington (US), were used. The diagnosis was standardised in a medical framework so that a group of people deemed to suffer the 'disease' schizophrenia was identified at each centre.

The IPSS established reliability of the diagnosis of schizophrenia (World Health Organisation 1979), but did not even attempt to establish cross-cultural validity of 'schizophrenia' – as measured by the PSE – as an illness, or even to establish the validity of the 'phenomena' on which the diagnosis was based. But the project proceeded as if it did do both these things. In keeping with a bio-medical model of illness, the next step in the IPSS was to follow-up the patients who had been identified as 'schizophrenic' in order to determine their prognoses. On the whole, the outcome of patients from (industrially) underdeveloped countries was superior to that in the (industrially developed) west, although, of course, the patients in western countries had more thorough psychiatric treatment and after-care. The methodology of the IPSS, as a cross-cultural study, has been seriously criticised, notably by Kleinman (1977):

> . . . it starts from a category fallacy which significantly limits its value as a study of cultural influences on mental illness. Its strength comes from reifying a narrowly defined syndrome affecting patients in nine separate cultural locations, but that is also its weakness. It is unable to systematically examine the impact of cultural factors on schizophrenia, since its methodology has ruled out the chief cultural determinants.
>
> (1977: 4)

However, the basic tool of the IPSS, the PSE (Wing *et al.* 1974), has been used in several cultures (Orley and Wing 1979; Okasha and Ashour 1981; Swartz *et al.* 1985), regardless of its lack of cross-cultural validity.

British research

Today, psychiatric research into what are called 'ethnic issues' continues at a rather alarming rate in Britain considering that, if anything, services for black and Asian communities are getting worse. The array of 'research findings' on ethnic issues are mainly concerned with counting the numbers of people given various diagnoses in what are termed 'epidemiological' surveys. As noted above (on p. 33), one of the main issues focuses on the over-representation of black people deemed 'schizophrenic'. As with research into other 'ethnic issues', successive surveys have made similar statistical conclusions but not really advanced knowledge about the basic findings or come up with any useful suggestions on improving clinical practice. Apart from the study by Parkman and colleagues (1997) quoted above (p. 34) (although this study was grossly inadequate in merely touching the surface of a vast problem) there have been no studies published in professional journals that draw on the experience of black patients (from their viewpoints) or their views about diagnosis and treatment. Nor, of course, have there been any studies of racism in the psychiatric system except for the study (quoted on p. 35) by Lewis and colleagues (1990) that I have already pointed out was flawed. So what is wrong?

Kuller (1999) has pointed out that good epidemiological studies 'progress from descriptive to analytic to experimental epidemiology and then to studies of effectiveness leading to prevention ' (1999: 897). Eaton and Harrison (2000) have pointed out that the lack of progress in British epidemiological psychiatric research into ethnic issues resembles what Kuller terms 'circular epidemiology', which is the continuation of a particular line of research after having established something beyond reasonable doubt. In my view, this has happened because researchers are unwilling or unable to question their methodology or test out hypotheses that may question dogmatically held ideologies. As Kuller puts it 'a new hypothesis for which there is lack of substantial prior data is unlikely to be successful in terms of peer review' (1999: 897), and hence unlikely to attract funding. I believe that (epidemiological) research into ethnic issues is stuck in a rut because researchers cannot or will not question the dogma of traditional diagnostic categorization; look for ways of analysis (of mental health problems) based on anything but western cultural concepts; shift from their adherence to the biomedical model that reduces the complexity of the human condition to consideration of 'illness' and 'normality'; and look at new ideas from service users and other stakeholders with an interest in the practice of psychiatry and mental health services. The question must be asked as to the usefulness of all this research and what the real (hidden) agenda may be. Why this apparent relentless search after better (*sic*) ways of diagnosing when the system of diagnosis itself is not being questioned? Why carry on counting 'schizophrenics'? Some discussion of the place of research in the total psychiatric picture may be helpful to the reader.

In our society today it is the written word that is generally accepted as the basis for knowledge, in particular words written in books and accredited journals which are well reviewed by important (*sic*) people. So when professionals talk of 'evidence-based practice' the only *evidence* that is taken as valid are papers written in these journals. What service users say about the services, diagnostic habits, and the effects of therapy, is not 'evidence'. And when a paper is published, the more professors there are on the editorial board of the journal, then the more power the papers in that journal carry. On the face of it there seems to be value in published work being vetted by one's peers, and in accepting that papers *should* carry power when they are subject to 'peer review'. And of course 'peer review' is considered to be the gold standard for approving research grants too. In suggesting a different view, I shall merely present two true stories and let the readers draw conclusions about hidden agendas.

A black psychiatrist was invited to work at a prestigious institute in south London in the late 1990s to study the issues around diagnosis of schizophrenia among black people. A joint paper was written by a white colleague quoting the black colleague's findings drawing the conclusion that diagnoses made by him were similar to those in case notes. (What diagnosis of schizophrenia means of course is a mute point when we consider the racist background of its development and the institutional racism of psychiatry today.) However, when the black colleague, by then resident abroad, saw a draft of the paper he found that (in his view) the data had been distorted in its presentation; the way he saw the data was that his diagnoses had been at variance with those in case notes. He wanted the paper changed. He was very surprised to hear that it had already been peer reviewed and accepted for the *British Journal of Psychiatry*! Now the punch line to this story is that when the paper was changed to reflect the correct findings, the peer reviewers started to quibble. It seemed that there was pressure to ensure that a great degree of variance in diagnosis was not presented in a publication. A compromise paper was later published.

The second story is about getting funding for research from the research committee connected with the secure (forensic) hospitals. In 1997 I was involved in applying for funding for a project to survey and evaluate the views of black service users who had been patients in a secure hospital. In spite of having the support of the hospital staff concerned (which was not easy) and the support of black staff within the body that dealt with the application, the proposal was turned down on the basis of 'peer review'. When I enquired about the reasons for the rejection, I found that, although the project was about service user views, no service user had been asked to review the project. Worse still there were neither service users nor black people on the panel that made decisions on the allocation of funds for research projects. I felt strongly enough to complain to the government minister in charge of mental health about the bias involved in research using taxpayers' money but got nowhere because it seems that the government does not interfere in medical research!

These stories illustrate the political nature of how psychiatric research is commissioned and how papers – research papers – get published. Of course the two are related because the more one gets published the more likely one is to get funded for research. The research and publication field today is highly competitive and often driven by economic gain for vested interests. If there are issues around race that appear to challenge psychiatry or the interests of prestigious university departments or the status of individuals, the question of publication is fraught; and the same can be said about getting funds for such research. The tragedy to my mind is that black people – researchers – are increasingly involved in maintaining this type of institutional racism. When several years ago, I protested to the civil servant at the Department of Health who was concerned with the allocation of funding for what I and other black professionals considered to be a flawed research project into 'psychosis' among black people, I was told that the project was 'alright' because a black registrar (junior doctor) was involved. But since then this type of research with black people's names attached have multiplied. More recently in 1993, another black professional and I were invited to serve on an advisory committee at the Department of Health in order to review a research project into deliberate self-harm among Asian women. The project put up by an Asian doctor for funding by the Department of Health envisaged assessments for clinical depression. When we (the two black people) wanted the project changed so that a social and cultural dimension was included alongside the medical approach proposed, we were both dropped from the committee and the research went ahead.

The main problem about psychiatric research in the field of ethnicity is that a complex field is being researched using telescopes that examine minutiae often determined by what researchers hope to find. In scientific terms, hard data which are useful in practice are very difficult to come by because the ways of research into ethnic issues are seriously flawed, essentially being too narrow-minded and reductionist. The fundamental problems of cross-cultural research, including the effect of racism in influencing judgements that go to make diagnoses, have not been addressed. Further, the tools used to measure 'culture', 'racism', etc., are far too narrow to yield useful information; in fact the 'information' that sometimes comes out when tools that are inappropriate to the task are used is misleading. Cross-cultural research today is often misdirected and misconceived – and generally far too timid (in being afraid to challenge vested interest) and unimaginative. The need to research institutional racism is not being tackled, possibly for political reasons. Notwithstanding the difficulties and problems, I believe that research into issues of race and culture ('ethnic issues') in the mental health field is necessary. But the tools must change and the agenda needs to be clarified. Possible ways forward are considered in Chapter 5.

Summary

The presence of black and Asian people in the UK has a very long history but it has become more evident during the past fifty years. The black presence in Britain is closely tied up with British conquests overseas – 'we are here because you were there'. The changing face of racism can be summarised by the terms used to describe the black presence: the 'Colour Problem' of the 1950s gave way to the 'Immigration Problem' of the 1970s and the 'Refugee Problem' of the 1990s. It is often said that Britain is committed to multiculturalism and cultural plurality is the ideal for British society. But the biggest barrier to multiculturalism, namely racism, has not been tackled adequately and all too often this failure is covered up with talk about 'culture' and more recently 'creed'. Although the ways in which racism is manifested and the extent of it may vary from place to place, racism as a barrier to multi-culturalism is evident all over Europe.

Ethnic issues in psychiatry and the mental health services have been evident for over fifteen years. The issues in the UK are probably replicated in most, if not all, European countries. The main issue for psychiatry is the over-diagnosis of schizophrenia among black people, but there are also issues for other professional groups in the mental health field and for the disciplines of counselling and psychotherapy. Research on ethnic issues in the mental health field continues but without apparently getting much further into understanding how racism can be addressed or cultural sensitivity brought into being. It is evident that the research agenda and methodology used in investigating matters to do with race and culture need to be fundamentally revised.

Chapter 2

Responding to racism, addressing culture

In this chapter I use the term 'black' in a 'political' or general sense to include Asian and other minority ethnic communities affected adversely by racism. The struggle against racism has not been easy. In the mental health field the response to the problems identified as 'ethnic issues' has been diverse and variable. In the UK there has emerged a 'black voluntary sector' attempting to provide services that aim to meet the needs of black (and Asian) people, but far too often projects have become corrupted or seduced into ineffectiveness. Attempts have been made in the statutory sector to address some of the problems – although these have been sporadic and often unsustained – usually by instituting training courses for staff and consulting with service users. The accounts in this chapter are a mixture of observations and analysis of information in the public domain, and personal views and experiences. The latter are based largely on what I have seen, heard about and experienced, backed up by efforts that I have made over the years in keeping up with what goes on in the field. References I make to Europe and countries in North America are sporadic and inconsistent because my own contacts and experience outside Britain are limited.

Struggle against racism

Racism has always been a problem for black people in Britain. They have struggled against it on two inter-connected fronts. First in direct confrontation by challenging racism at various levels – as prejudiced behaviour, racial attacks and institutional racism. Second, by getting together in various ways to support each other, forming self-help groups, etc. But none of this has been plain sailing. Stated intentions of the government to counteract racism have not usually been translated into changes on the ground. The rhetoric of black leaders has often not been matched by action when they achieve positions from where they can take action. But yet there has been progress. In general my feeling of the change over the past twenty years is that the struggle has changed some-what from a struggle by black people with little general support, to one where black and white are on the same side – more-or-less. In the mental health field too the struggle appears now (at the time of writing) to being honestly pursued for *the first time* (in my experi-ence) not just by black users of mental health services, their carers, and some black professionals, but by politicians and civil servants in charge of mental health services. Yet, changes are far too slow and far too often impeded by tokenism and rhetoric that is not backed up by action.

In the 1950s and 1960s, black people began to develop com-munity groups, usually serving a social function for black people who felt excluded from mainstream. What gradually came to be called the 'black voluntary sector' further expanded in the 1970s. But funding was always a great problem. In the 1980s the black voluntary sector was given a boost when urban programmes of local authorities, especially the Greater London Council in London, supported minority groups directly. From the early 1980s onwards, the black voluntary sector has been an important support for the struggle against racism. In the late 1980s (when the Greater London Council was abolished) many local authorities cut funding of local minority groups of all kinds. So the minority ethnic groups that have emerged since then have depended much more on grass roots support than earlier groups did – in some ways a healthier position to that in the 1980s when, with govern-ment funding, some groups had developed a 'grant-aided mentality rather than one of advocacy and grassroots campaigning' (Wenham 1993: 9).

In their book *Policing the Crisis* Hall and colleagues (1978) describe how the 1970s in Britain saw rising publicity being given to street crimes in British cities fostering the impression of 'a dramatic and unexpected epidemic of "mugging"' (1978: 17). Black com-munities ('immigrants') were openly blamed for these crimes by the press leading to a tightening of social control being exercised on black people. More generally, social problems were blamed on the post-war immigration of 'coloured' people and an Immigration Act was introduced in 1971 that virtually ended the immigration of people from Asia, Africa and the Caribbean. This immigration law re-enforced the perception of black people as a problem, particularly by the police. Overt racism was rife on the streets and in employment. In 1976, a Race Relations Act was introduced making certain types of racial discrimination an offence (Home Office 1976). In 1980 and 1981, Britain's first inner-city riots occurred (see Solomos *et al.* 1982) in which mainly black African-Caribbean youth took to the streets causing disturbances reminiscent of 'race riots' in the US. The (then) Tory government appointed Lord Scarman to investigate the causes of these disturbances.

1980s and 1990s

The report by Lord Scarman (Home Office 1981) denied the existence of institutional racism and blamed the riots on a mixture of the attitudes of young black people, racial disadvantage suffered by them, and the inexperience of police officers. According to Lord Scarman, young black people 'living much of their lives on the streets . . . are brought into contact with the police who appear to them as visible symbols of the authority of a society that has failed to bring them its benefits' (1981: 11). The remedies recommended by Scarman consisted of positive action to meet (what were called) 'the special problems and needs of ethnic minorities' (1981: 108) and action to remedy discrimination in housing, education, etc. As a result, there were active efforts to promote religious and cultural identities of ethnic minority groups and some authorities also encouraged psycho-educational approaches, such as racial awareness training for white people – racial awareness training being an approach that addressed personal prejudice rather than institutional processes (as discussed on pp. 49–51). Looked at with hindsight, this report set back progress in tackling racism (Bourne 2001), by presenting disadvantage as 'some sort of handicap' (2001: 11) suffered by black people. Scarman 'effectively reduced (objective) institutional racism to (individual) black perception, on the one hand, and personal (white) prejudice, on the other, and so shifted the object of anti-racist struggle from the state to the individual, from changing society to changing people, from improving the lot of whole black communities, mired in poverty and racism to improving the lot of black individuals' (2001: 12).

In my experience in the mental health field, racial awareness training of the 1980s was ineffective for two reasons. First, people attending racial awareness training courses often shrugged them off as not applicable to them since they were not racist; and second, those 'trained' often felt absolved from having to do anything further about racism. I well recall social workers returning to work after such training, confident that they were no longer 'racist'. Looking back on the post-Scarman era in London, the impression left was that racism was interpreted as being 'prejudice plus power' so that the remedies lay in race-based equality policies that substituted black faces for white (hopefully in positions of power) rather than changing structures of society that supported and promoted such inequalities (Bourne 2001), and in attempting to induce people to change their attitudes (i.e. drop their prejudices). At an institutional level, equal opportunity policies that addressed race inequality in employment practice were seen as the answer in the long run.

London in the 1980s saw 'a flurry of reports, working groups and conferences on local authority strategies to combat racial disadvantage' (Sivanandan 1985: 22). But, if anything, racial disadvantage in housing, unemployment and schooling got worse. Racially motivated violence was rife and resulted in several deaths of black people (Gordon 1986). Deaths of black people in police custody were reported regularly – and largely ignored by the media and government. In spite of concerns voiced by the then Home Secretary following a Home Office study in 1981 into the incidence of racial attacks across the British Isles, six years later the Commission for Racial Equality reported no drop in their incidence (Commission for Racial Equality 1987). The proportion of black people in prison rose steadily and by 1990 it was 15.5 per cent for men and 25.8 per cent for women (Institute of Race Relations 1991), but according to a report issued by the Runnymede Trust in 1990, racism in the criminal justice system 'was largely unrecognised and undocumented by organisations supposedly concerned with the advancement of civil liberties, the protection of rights and the achievement of justice' (Shallice and Gordon 1990: 55).

In 1993, a young black man was murdered in south London. Although many black people felt that the police failed to investigate the murder adequately, calls on the (then) Home Secretary to institute a public inquiry were rejected. However, the incoming Labour Government of 1997 did just that. The inquiry, under the chairmanship of Sir William Macpherson, attracted much media attention during the hearings and even more attention when its report was published in February 1999 (Home Department 1999) highlighting widespread racism – not just within the police but also in all public institutions. Suddenly the need to counteract racism in all public bodies was on the government agenda and, for the first time, the emphasis was on institutional racism, defined in the report as:

> The collective failure of an organisation to provide an appropriate and professional service to people because of their colour, culture or ethnic origin. It can be seen or detected in processes, attitudes and behaviour which amount to discrimination through unwitting prejudice, ignorance, thoughtlessness and racist stereotyping which disadvantages minority ethnic people.
>
> (1999: 28)

The (then) Secretary of State for Home Affairs (Jack Straw), who commissioned the Macpherson inquiry, spoke strongly of the need to counteract racism in all public bodies. Ethnic recruitment and retention policies were set for the police force, a new definition of a 'racial incident' was created to oblige the police to investigate racially motivated violence, and, most importantly (although after some hesitation), the government brought in an amendment to the Race Relations Act 1976 (Home Office 2001) extending the scope of anti-racist legislation and making it a statutory obligation for public bodies to actively promote racial equality. In noting with concern the disproportionately large numbers of black young men being stopped and searched by the police in major British cities, the Macpherson Report recommended that police officers should provide reasons in writing for carrying out the 'stop and search' procedure.

Two years after the Macpherson Report, considerable doubts were being voiced on the effectiveness of the post-Macpherson changes and actions (Bourne 2001). And now (at the time of writing) statistics issued by the Home Office (2002a) suggest that racism in the police force may have worsened since the Macpherson Report was issued. According to these statistics, 'ethnic minorities are over-represented in those dismissed or resigning from the Police and Prison Service'; and in comparing figures for 2001/2002 with those for 2000/2001, the number of recorded stops and searches rose by 8% for white people and 30% for black people and 40% for Asian in the Metropolitan Police Area (MPS) . . . [although] the proportion of those arrested following a stop and search remained unchanged at 13% for white people, 17% for black people and 15% for Asians.

(Home Office 2002a: 14)

Notwithstanding these ominous signs of a worsening of racism, the Macpherson Report was clearly a watershed in the struggle against racism in society at large. Perhaps for the first time, black people felt that racism was being recognised as a problem for all of society and one that the Government was determined to address. But this determination did not carry through very far into the new millennium.

2000 plus

In the spring and early summer of 2001, violence broke out in three northern cities in England – Bradford, Burnley and Oldham – in which both Asian youths and white people were separately involved in skirmishes with police. An analysis of race in Britain in an eminent British newspaper (*The Observer*) concluded in its editorial (2001) that this was not a flash in the pan but a result of deliberate activities of the (racist and fascist) British National Party in the context of 'decades of simmering resentment' (2001: 1). Several official inquires were held into what were soon dubbed 'race riots' but unfortunately the reports did not appear for nearly six months – by which time the 'race' context had changed dramatically.

On September 11, 2001 there was an attack on the twin towers of the World Trade Center in New York – an attack attributed to the work of 'Islamic' terrorists. A 'war against terrorism' was launched by the US supported by the UK. Anti-terrorist legislation limiting human rights was rushed through both countries and checks based on racial profiling (i.e. identifying people as suspects on the basis of their apparent racial origin) meant that brown-skinned and black-skinned people were targeted as terrorist suspects (Monbiot 2002). The effect of all this on public perceptions of racial issues was confusing and problematic. A study of bias crimes in the US after September 11 found that 96 per cent of documented attacks targeted south Asians (Krishna 2002). I believe that the effects were even more widespread.

A few days before the main report on the 2001 riots, the Cantle Report (Independent Review Team 2001), was released, the Secretary of State for Home Affairs, David Blunkett, pre-empted its publication with some extraordinary statements in which (as a renowned journalist put it) 'Going straight for the extreme, he listed all the worst aspects of religions and customs [of ethnic minorities] as if these things were everyday occurrences. . . . And nothing about the white community and its obligation to reconsider the changed nature of Britishness' (Toynbee 2001: 16). By talking of classes in citizenship and the English language for immigrants he seemed to question the loyalty of ethnic minorities at a time when the country was said to be 'at war' with 'terrorists'. He muddied the debate on race, confusing 'race' with 'religion' and making no distinction between recent immigrants and third-generation Asian youths who were involved in the 'race riots'. The change from the approach of his predecessor Jack Straw (see p. 50) could not have been greater.

The Cantle Report draws attention to the need to avoid – and counteract – segregation of racial groups and promote 'community cohesion' through greater contact between people from different cultural backgrounds. The report appears to blame the Asian populations involved in the riots for this 'segregation' – or at least the government and some media take this as the message of the report. But what is not even mentioned in the report is that segregation results from policies – and lack of policies – that condone and encourage 'white flight' (the tendency of white people to move away from an area when black and Asian people move into it), the dumping of Asians in 'sink estates' by local councils, and racial harassment (Phillips 2001). Two other reports on the 2001 riots commissioned locally rather than being commissioned by central government, one on Oldham (Oldham Independent Panel 2001) and one on Burnley (Burnley Task Force 2001), take a very different stance to that taken by the Cantle Report. They highlight the employment discrimination against Asians, the need to ensure racially mixed housing schemes, the fact that racial tension is exploited by organised racists, poverty, and entrenched racist views in the society. Significantly, what has been taken up by the media and government ministers is the apparent support in the Cantle Report for David Blunkett's comments (noted above).

Blunkett has taken matters further by announcing, in an immigration white paper (Home Office 2002b), that the government is considering an oath of allegiance for immigrants, and issuing (what he called) 'advice' to Asian people not to seek marriage partners from the Asian subcontinent (Blackstock 2002). And, in the course of defending his statements, Blunkett has worsened the situation even further by appearing to confuse (in his statements) arranged marriages with forced marriages and talking of preventing female genital mutilation.

Overall, the Cantle Report, taken with David Blunkett's statements, seems to set out a major shift in government policy on race away from that instituted after the Macpherson Report (Home Department 1999). While the struggle against racism was seen in 1999 as one for British society as a whole, less than three years later a 'them and us' approach has again been introduced. Instead of leading the discussions in line with commitments made in 2000 by the Labour government to 'creating one nation . . . where every colour is a good colour . . . racism is unacceptable and counteracted . . . and racial diversity celebrated' (Home Office 2000: 1), black and Asian people are again being asked to prove their loyalty and their adherence to 'British values', and Asians (not white people) are being asked to marry people from within the country! The 'race relations' clock has being set back thirty years. Clearly, if this new agenda is pursued the struggle against racism would have to change its approaches too.

The exacerbation of racist feelings in Britain since September 11 may well have brought about the change of heart in government circles. The pervasiveness of this change is illustrated by a personal experience. On 21 September 2001, I attended (and spoke at) a meeting organised by black and Asian social workers in a west London borough. In talking with the Director of Social Services for the borough during the coffee break, I mentioned the need for supporting black and Asian voluntary organisation in the borough (in which the minority ethnic population was in excess of 30 per cent). To my astonishment his spontaneous response was 'It's very difficult now, since the September 11 attack'. Noticing my surprise he went on 'it's not me, it's that people wouldn't like it', and he then moved on quickly. So, with 'Islam' being identified as something dangerous and 'foreign' in the US and Britain, all black people are being seen as 'foreign' and suspect. In other words, hostility towards people perceived as Muslims is being merged with racism based on skin colour, 'a backlash against people who look different – Asian in particular' as the former Chairman of the Commission of Racial Equality (Singh 2001: 9) puts it. Racism expressed in cultural language has graduated into racism expressed in the language of religion or creed. And sure enough, a BBC radio series on 'Race, Culture and Creed' began on 26 December 2001 by discussing the proposition 'Religion not race is the major obstacle to a multicultural society' (BBC 2001).

Responses in the mental health field

As in the general struggle against racism (as discussed in the preceding section), there are two strands in the struggle for change in the mental health field. First, there is the direct approach in highlighting injustices and deficiencies in the services, and second, the development of projects by and for black and minority ethnic communities, including self-help projects. The latter is of course inseparable from the former and is represented by initiatives for change in both the statutory sector and the black voluntary sector. I attempt in this chapter to describe the former in terms of a struggle that is inseparable from the struggle to bring about a culturally sensitive service. Then I make some comments about some innovative projects in the mental health field. These are not necessarily the main projects around or the best of the bunch – they just happen to be ones I know (or have known) quite well.

Highlighting issues has not been straightforward; it is sometimes a double-edged sword. For example, when the high rates at which second-generation black people were being given the 'schizophrenia' label became evident (Chapter 1) the medical establishment and the media took it up in the context of discussions about the black presence in Britain. An eminent psychiatrist from the Institute of Psychiatry quoted the so-called high 'incidence' of schizophrenia among black people as evidence that 'something had gone dreadfully wrong for the Caribbean second generation' (Ballantyne 1988: 6). An immunological/virus theory was proposed as an explanation for this 'high incidence' (of schizophrenia among black people) by a professor of psychiatry from Nottingham University in a BBC television programme – a programme actually *called* 'Black Schizophrenia' – broadcast on 13 March 1989 (the spurious basis for this theory is given below). In this programme, based on a paper by Harrison *et al.* (1988), schizophrenia among

black people was discussed against visual images of rioting by
black youth, and the 'virus theory' was discussed against images of
West Indians coming off boats (see Fernando 1989). The
suggestion that 'black schizophrenia' was associated with violence
and immigration was obvious. The programme was objected to by
Mind (the National Association for Mental Health) and the
Transcultural Psychiatry Society in a joint letter to the Director of
the BBC, and there was correspondence (Fernando 1989; Brightwell 1989) in the official BBC journal *The Listener* about the
programme and a supporting article (Tilby 1989).

The background to the 'virus theory' for schizophrenia is worth
noting. Two studies of the 1957 influenza epidemic (Mednick *et al.*
1989; O'Callaghan *et al.* 1991) found an association between viral
infection in women and a diagnosis of schizophrenia in their
offspring but data from other studies (Kendell and Kemp 1989;
Selten and Slaets 1994; Susser *et al.* 1994; Torrey *et al.* 1988) failed
to detect such an association. The tenuous evidence from the two
positive studies (ignoring the negative ones) was linked up with the
possibility that perinatal virus infection *may* have led to an
immunological dysfunction (King and Cooper 1989) that in turn
may have led to brain damage leading to schizophrenia – all
speculation! Then a number of researchers (e.g. Wing 1989;
Harrison 1990; Eagles 1991; Wessely *et al.* 1991; Harrison *et al.*
1997) quoted this immunological–virus theory or a variation of it
in order to explain away the relatively high likelihood of young
British-born black men being diagnosed as 'schizophrenic'. More
recently, an association between schizophrenia and the 1957
influenza epidemic has been firmly rejected (Crow and Done 1992;
Cannon *et al.* 1996), although some psychiatrists (e.g. Adams and
Kendell 1996) try to cling to the (now discredited) hypothesis that
was based on such an alleged association – namely that maternal
virus infection is a cause of schizophrenia in offspring. The alacrity
with which institutional psychiatry, represented by eminent British
psychiatrists, grabbed at the virus theory shows the powerful need
for psychiatry to protect its current ways of thinking (and hence
working), even at the expense of perpetuating the racism which it
has inherited from the past.

While psychiatry as an institution was vigorously avoiding any
reference to racism, or even to any doubt that psychiatric
methodology may be influenced by institutional racism, anecdotal
evidence from black service users indicated that psychiatry itself

was dreadfully wrong in some way. Gradually total denial was replaced by admission of 'cultural' problems. Yet, whenever training was instituted to address (what were usually called) 'cultural' issues, the schemes were generally implemented half heartedly and without much financial support – and they carefully avoided addressing issues around racism. But gradually psychiatry as an institution accepted that 'race' might play some part in producing inequities in the way psychiatry was practised. Yet, the way in which a report into deaths of black people at Broadmoor Hospital (Special Hospitals Service Authority 1993) was handled exemplifies the problems of addressing racism in psychiatry. This report was commissioned by the Special Hospitals Service Authority that governed all special – or high security – hospitals at the time, Broadmoor Hospital then being one of four such hospitals in the UK. The report highlighted racism as a major factor in the events leading to the deaths and recommended 'further research into the diagnosis of schizophrenia in Afro-Caribbeans . . . [and the monitoring of] patterns of diagnosis among minority ethnic groups in the special hospital system' (1993: 52). The hospital authorities rejected the report and the Special Hospitals Service Authority ignored it, even failing to print sufficient numbers of copies of the report to meet the demand from the public. I know this because when I telephoned the Special Hospitals Service Authority for copies of the report a few weeks after its publication, I was told that it was no longer available and would not be reprinted. The press largely ignored its findings and the television services totally ignored it. However, reports that seemed to imply that black people were particularly dangerous (because of 'schizophrenia'), such as the Clunis Inquiry Report (North East Thames Regional Health Authority and South East Thames Regional Health Authority 1994), were taken up in a big way by all the media with pictures of the alleged dangerous (black) persons.

Striving for change

1980s

Endeavours by black people, professionals and the general public alike, to highlight the racial injustices within British psychiatry and psychology took off vigorously in the 1980s. Also, black and Asian people began to get together in the 1980s to develop services for their communities outside the statutory mental health sector. The highlighting of the issues may be connected with changes that occurred within the Transcultural Psychiatry Society in the early 1980s – changes that resulted in this society taking a lead in publicising race and culture issues appertaining to psychiatric practice (see pp. 67–8). As the high rates of compulsory detention of black people and their liability to be diagnosed as 'schizo-phrenic' became substantiated by research publications (Chapter 1), concern about possible racism within psychiatry was high-lighted. The Mental Health Act Commission, a government inspectorate that was put in place after a new Mental Health Act came on line in 1983, took up the issues at an official level through its reports (Mental Health Act Commission 1987, 1991). Also, its visiting teams were instructed to take up these issues during the course of official visits to individual mental health facilities, although I know from personal observation (while a member of the Mental Health Act Commission from 1986 until 1995) that the degree to which this was implemented varied considerably. Since members of the Mental Health Act Commission, 'commissioners', clearly did not fully appreciate the importance of race and culture issues for ordinary patients, training in race and culture for commissioners was put on by the Mental Health Act Commission. A lobby developed within the Mental Health Act Commission centred on what became officially its Standing Committee on Race and Culture. The problems that resulted within that body illustrate the nature of the struggle that often takes place (usually behind closed doors) in many organisations connected with mental health. Some of the happenings within the Mental Health Act Commission (in which I was involved) are worth presenting here.

I joined the Mental Health Act Commission in 1986. In 1989, a new Chairman was appointed to head the organisation – a barrister with a reputation for radical politics and a forthright approach. The 'working party on black and ethnic minorities' which I chaired at the time, was renamed the 'National Standing Committee on Race and Culture', as all working parties were renamed 'National Standing Committees' (NSCs). In October 1989, all commissioners had a memorandum from the Commission Chairman stating that in future all national standing committees will be chaired by persons appointed by him. When the names of the selected chairpersons were announced a few days later they turned out to be the people already in post except for the NSC on Race and Culture, which was given a new chairperson – a white man who had previously not been involved in the committee at all. I then undertook a long struggle which involved (a) obtaining legal advice on the applicability of the Race Relation Act to the action of the Commission Chairman and making this known to members of the Central Policy Committee (CPC), the governing body of the Mental Health Act Commission at that time; (b) appraising individual members of the CPC of my treatment by the Commission Chairman; and (c) making the issues (as I saw it) known unofficially to persons at the Department of Health. At the end of this, the Commission chairman changed his earlier action and nominated me as the Chairman of the NSC on Race and Culture.

The Commission chairman seemed to think that this private resolution was adequate and invited me to 'have a drink'. However, in my view nothing had been done to preclude a repetition of similar racist actions within the Commission. Institutional practice had to change. Under threats of public exposure if he did not, the Chairman, negotiating through an intermediary, agreed to support an official policy for the Mental Health Act Commission that would render future racist actions unsustainable and ensure monitoring of staffing arrangements within the Commission from an anti-racist viewpoint. The policy – 'Race Policy' – was agreed by the Commission and published in the fourth and fifth commission reports (Mental Health Act Commission 1991; 1993). I believe that this policy was a landmark in the work of the Commission. But the question at the time was 'would it last?' It certainly helped later when the NSC on Race and Culture, in the course of monitoring the Race Policy, demanded a proper ethnic mix of membership of the CPC, and got it.

The Race Policy itself was revised just before I left the Commission in 1995 and renamed 'The Policy on Race and Culture' (Mental Health Act Commission 1995: 210–12). However, the seventh commission report (Mental Health Act Commission 1997), issued after I left the Mental Health Act Commission, does not refer to a policy on race at all but merely to the Commission having identified 'three target areas' as a 'focus during visits', namely ethnic monitoring, interpreters and racial harassment (1997: 158). Gone, it seems, is the need to keep the Commission 'free of discriminatory practices on racial grounds' (Mental Health Act Commission 1995: 212) and monitor the actions of the Commission itself for institutional racism. A wider consideration of my experiences as a member of the Mental Health Act Commission, including more details of the issues given above, are described elsewhere (Fernando 1996). The organisation of the work of the Mental Health Act Commission has changed considerably since 1995. My impression is that it is now seen as being relatively weak with respect to highlighting issues of a fundamental nature. It would seem that the anti-racist approach epitomised by the Race Policy that was operational from 1991 until 1995 has been abandoned in favour of a 'culture-sensitivity' and 'equal-opportunity' approach. Perhaps a sign of the times even before the changes in government policy envisaged by David Blunkett (described pp. 52–3).

Several psychiatrists, both black and white, were involved early on in promoting an anti-racist agenda in mental health services. Many of these people were members of the Transcultural Psychiatry Society and meetings of this society during the 1980s were in the forefront of the struggle against racism in psychiatry. Dr (now Professor) Sashi Sashidharan (of Indian origin), Dr Aggrey Burke (of African-Caribbean origin) and Dr (now Professor) Roland Littlewood (white-English origin) were all colleagues in the struggle during those years. At the level of campaigning, Yvonne Christie and others lobbied the (then Tory) government for many years and indeed worked with its task force on mental health in the early 1990s. Meanwhile people struggled at grass roots promoting services, Errol Francis and Tanzeem Ahmed come to mind. In the field of child and adolescent psychiatry, Dr Annie Lau (of Chinese origin) wrote and lectured in promoting a culturally sensitive approach in family therapy. Ground work, done within some statutory organisations such as the Central Council for Education and Training of Social Workers (CCETSW), was significant at the time too. Naina Patel was prominent at CCETSW, and it is salutary to recall that CCETSW's work on anti-racism led to a backlash of sorts in the late 1980s leading to its eventual replacement with a less radical organisation.

The 1980s saw the advent of innovative services such as Nafsiyat (described briefly later in this chapter), a psychotherapy service for ethnic minorities founded by Jafar Kareem, a psychotherapist of

Indian origin. However, few agencies, and least of all the government got very far in addressing the problems that black people faced when they accessed mental health services and the serious problems of race and culture within psychiatry. But there was progress in related areas such as developing equal opportunities in employment and even sometimes an understanding of institutional racism within mental health services, reflected for example in the content of successive reports of the Mental Health Act Commission (1991, 1993, 1995). Also in the 1980s health projects targeting black and ethnic minorities were coming on line (see 'Initiatives in mental health service provision' below).

There were many conferences in the 1980s, sometimes attended by government ministers. Although voices were being raised about the exclusion from mental health services of Asian people because of racism and the cultural insensitivity of psychiatry, for example in *Illness or Distress* (Beliappa 1991) and *A Cry for Change* (Webb-Johnson, 1991), the main issues highlighted were the high levels of compulsory detention ('sectioning') of black people and the apparent over-diagnosis of schizophrenia among black patients. Although both these matters should have been of concern to psychiatrists, the Royal College of Psychiatrists (the professional organisation of British psychiatrists) seemed impervious to any representations, denying that any problem existed. However, towards the end of the 1980s, under pressure from some of its black members and the Mental Health Act Commission, the College established a committee to look into services for ethnic minorities chaired by an ex-president of the College, Professor Rawnsley. This committee failed to agree on a final report but some indication of the 'leadership' provided to that committee may be discerned from the following anecdote. In a BBC radio programme *Face the Facts* broadcast in September 1987, Rawnsley (1987) claimed that 'research evidence' showed that black people were over-represented among people diagnosed as 'schizophrenic' because (compared to white people) they were more violent, more likely to indulge in criminal activity, and less compliant in taking medication. And he went on to give his opinion that black people's alleged predisposition to violence was 'culturally determined behaviour'. The significance of Rawnsley's public statements was that there was no research at that time into ethnic differences in criminal activity among patients or into their compliance with medication; while the only research that had looked at ethnic differences in the likelihood of violence among patients (Harrison *et al.* 1984) had actually shown the opposite to what Rawnsley stated, a fact verified by the researchers speaking on the same radio programme. There can be no better example of the power of stereotypes being held *in spite of* evidence to the contrary (as 'delusions' are said to hold in psychopathology). As the 1980s wore on little seemed to have changed as far as the ordinary practice of psychiatry and clinical psychology was concerned, and hence in the negative experiences suffered by black users of the mental health services.

1990s

The early 1990s saw increasing pressures on services and professionals working in them, accompanied by strenuous criticism of mental health services by users of the services and, for very different reasons (e.g. alleged risk of violence perpetrated by 'mental patients') by the public at large. Many professionals felt that they were blamed for what amounted to problems resulting from service deficiencies. The 'ethnic' scene in the British health services had changed considerably from that in the 1970s. Black people were a visible presence in many levels of the health professions and management – although still relatively poorly represented in its higher echelons – partly as a result of both the equal opportunities policies introduced in the 1980s and their own personal struggles against racism. In this context, the interest in race issues lapsed in the mid-1990s, possibly because there was a general feeling that having a fair number of black professionals in positions of influence represented 'change', in keeping with the post-Scarman era described earlier (see pp. 48–9). About that time ethnic monitoring was introduced into mental health services but it was not properly implemented. The attitudes around were a mixture of complacency among managers and the 'white establishment' coupled with disillusionment among black people, especially users of mental health services and thinking professionals (e.g. those within the Transcultural Psychiatry Society). In the early 1990s so-called development workers, who had been appointed in the late 1980s to address race and culture issues in health services and to develop appropriate services for ethnic minorities, were eased out of their commitments, usually by absorbing their work into mainstream services. Mainstreaming became, and still survives as, a euphemism for abolishing. Projects for black people found it more difficult to get funding, and some active projects were dismantled through mainstreaming. And so on. Although by then there were many policies supposed to counteract inequalities, generally speaking, the scene at grass roots was not changing much; having black faces at management level and in the professions was not resulting in changes at the level of 'patient care' or in the experience of service users. The apparent collusion of black professionals in failing to counter, or even in promoting racism was most marked in the field of institutional psychiatry, in forensic psychiatry in particular, and in the research agenda generated by prestigious institutions (see Chapter 1). The fundamental issues of institutionalised racism within the disciplines that inform mental health services were not even being touched.

The advent of a Labour government in Britain in June 1997 raised the hopes of many people for positive action in redressing various injustices, not least issues around racism. Paul Boateng, a black activist with a record of fighting racism in local government, was appointed as the minister in charge of mental health within the Department of Health. Boateng, a solicitor, had legally represented many black people on mental health review tribunals and so knew the score as far as black people's experiences with psychiatry were concerned. On appointment as a minister he claimed a commitment to counteract racism in mental health and the practice of psychiatry, but unfortunately failed to match rhetoric with action. Indeed, when the Department of Health announced its intentions to develop a framework for mental health services, it appeared to bypass Boating's assurances that racial inequities in mental health services and racism in psychiatric practice would be addressed. The 'external reference group' (ERG) that the Department of Health established for consultation (for the framework) was constructed in such a way that the voices of black people, especially service users from these communities, were marginalized. The matter came into the public domain with a letter to the Secretary of State (Minister) for Health, Frank Dobson, from sixteen mental health professionals involved in both the statutory and voluntary sectors. This letter, published in full in *Openmind* (Fernando 1998a) and referred to in national newspapers, included the following explanation of how the black voice had been sidestepped.

This has been done by a combination of (a) including in the groups many people of high status from prestigious bodies concerned with maintaining the status quo; (b) appointing very few Black and Asian people, mostly without experience of committee work, and some clearly token appointments of people not in a position to voice race and culture issues; and (c) not appointing people who have been in the forefront of advising on and developing strategies to counteract inequalities arising from these issues (some with an international eminence in these areas). We are surprised that a Labour Government which has stated a public commitment to counteract social exclusion should preside over a policy by one of its departments of practising exclusion.

(1998a: 15)

Clearly a black minister committed to oppose racism had been unable to prevent institutional racism in his own department. The National Service Framework for Mental Health that eventually emerged (Department of Health 1999) contained very little of any substance with regard to race and culture, and nothing that suggested action on racism although admitting that 'black and minority ethnic communities lack confidence in mental health services' (1999: 17)

Following the Macpherson Report (Home Department 1999) referred to earlier (see pp. 49–50), many public bodies, including the Department of Health, instituted audits of institutional racism. Many health authorities and social services departments began to promote training of their staff directed at counteracting racism and they seemed to focus particularly on mental health services. In September 2001 the Royal College of Psychiatrists appointed an external consultancy to carry out an independent review of institutional racism within the College structures (see Cox 2001); and two papers (Sashidharan 2001; Cox, 2001) in its official organ (*Psychiatric Bulletin*) attempted to open a debate on institutional racism within British psychiatry, making official something that had been debated outside the College for many years. The Commissioner for Mental Health (commonly called the 'mental health tsar') delegated Professor Sashidharan to develop a strategy for dealing with race and culture issues within mental health services. The significance of this is that, until this event, Professor Sashidharan had been marginalized by the government and the Royal College of Psychiatrists quite clearly because of his open criticism of racism within psychiatry and the College structures.

Refugees and asylum seekers

Since the 1980s, many of the newcomers to Britain who identify as being black, Asian or more generally of an 'ethnic minority' have been refugees and asylum seekers. Although facing similar problems to those faced by settled minority ethnic communities, these newcomers also present additional challenges for the mental health services such as problems with personal torture and political pressures. The media, and even the government, tend to focus on these newcomers as 'problems', just as black people had been seen as problems in earlier years. In fact much of the racism in the later 1990s, often overtly expressed, has taken the form of hostility to refugees and asylum seekers. Until the mid-1990s the idea that mental health services may have to address the needs of refugees was rejected at many levels. For example, I recall going to the Department of Health in late 1996 to ask about financial support in providing counselling services for refugees within an established service for ethnic minorities, only to be told that the Department of Health did not see the need for specific projects for refugees because they were 'not here to stay'.

A change that took place as a result of the change of government in 1997 was that, in spite of bringing in oppressive policies, such as the strategy of dispersing asylum seekers to various parts of the country and their detention in prison when they have committed no crime, the Labour Government encouraged and financed many services directed at relieving stresses suffered by refugees and asylum seekers. As a result, the late 1990s and the early years of the new millennium has seen a strong interest in developing mental health services that are appropriate and sensitive to the needs of refugees. So much so that 'refugee mental health' has almost become a bandwagon for researchers and trainers looking for funding. In my opinion, refugees should be seen as 'black and Asian' or belonging to 'minority ethnic' groups so that all the knowledge already available about the problems faced by these groups in receiving appropriate and just services can be accessed. Professionals involved in working with refugees need look no further than the transcultural psychiatry movement for information and approaches for their work. Re-inventing the wheel through conferences and research is not necessary; it is action to set up services that address cultural diversity and racism that is required.

Current scene

The extent to which changes in attitude since 11 September 2001 (to issues of 'race') will affect mental health services and psychiatry, is difficult to foresee. My impression is that, at the very least, the agenda for counteracting racism is now less of a priority for society as a whole, and hence more difficult to pursue *vis-à-vis* mental health services, than it was prior to September 11. Consequently, such an agenda must become *more* of a priority for black and Asian communities (including refugees and asylum seekers) in the UK and the rest of Europe. It is possible that the procedures already put in place, some of which have been described above (see p. 63), may be sufficient to carry forward the structural changes necessary for a start to be made in dismantling institutional racism in mental health and psychiatry. However, there is no panacea or short cut. There is no circumscribed 'good practice' answer, no ready-made 'new model' of psychiatry – indeed of mental health – that will suffice. However, ways forward are discernible and, with goodwill and perseverance, achievable. These will be discussed in Chapter 5, after transcultural perspectives on some aspects of mental health and the subtleties of racism have been explored, using concepts of stigma, power and discrimination, in Chapter 4.

There have been many conferences focusing on the need for change. The themes that have come up at conferences during the 1980s and 1990s are very clear (Box 2.1). First, current training instils a (quite unrealistic and 'racist') confidence in the superiority of the body of knowledge within psychiatry and psychology over that of knowledge about human beings evident in non-western cultures. Second, mental health assessments fail to allow for ideologies about life, approaches to life's problems, beliefs and feelings that come from non-western cultures. The causes of justified anger arising from racism in society are often not recognised because the black experience in society is not given credence, and eurocentric explanations derived from traditional psychiatry and

Box 2.1 Themes at conferences: issues

Training of professionals
Mental health assessments
'Therapy' and outcome
Alienation and exclusion

psychology are used to interpret problems that are essentially social and political. Stereotypical assumptions about black people or Asian people, or refugees, influence assessments that professionals make, 'treatments' that people are given, and so on. In the next chapter I take some of the arguments started here a little further. And in Chapter 5 I consider the sort of actions that may be practicable in the immediate future.

Europe

Mental health services in mainland European countries are generally organised very differently to those in the UK. In many of those countries, health care is usually funded by insurance systems rather than by the state, so it is difficult to compare the situation in mainland Europe with that in Britain (where services are based on a National Health Service funded by general taxation). Further, as a researcher in the mental health field (Watters 2002) states 'There is very little recent comparative material on mental health services in Europe, let alone specific information on services for migrant groups' (2002: 153). Finally there is very little information on the extent to which the disciplines of psychiatry and psychology on the European mainland address issues of race and culture.

The first attempt to get together a European network to discuss race and culture issues was a conference held in September 1991 in Rotterdam titled 'Mental Health and Multicultural Societies in the Europe of the Nineties'. A group of participants at that meeting met one year later and formed the 'Platform on Multi-Cultural Societies and Mental Health' under the aegis of the European section of the World Health Organisation. The meetings of this group, which I was privileged to belong to, have been in abeyance since September 1995. A second European conference 'Mental Health Race and Culture in Europe' was held in Bristol (UK) in April 1994 (Lucas 1994) but an intention of the organisers to repeat it has not materialised. Apart from the many books on issues of race and culture in mental health and psychiatry that have appeared in Britain (in English), the few books aimed at other European countries with contributions by professionals from minority ethnic communities ('black Europeans') in those countries include books by Linburg-Okken (1989) and Boedjarath and van Bekkum (1997) in The Netherlands, and by Salman and colleagues (1999) and Hegemann and Salman (2001) in Germany.

In reporting a limited survey of eighteen countries carried out in 1998, Watters (2002) states 'An overall impression is that in many European countries migrant groups [i.e. settled minority ethnic communities and recent arrivals as refugees or asylum seekers] have an entitlement to mental health care services but that these services are not designed to meet their needs' (2002: 167). However, Watters also reports an impression of substantial differences in the extent to which services have been developed for settled minority ethnic groups and for refugees: in some countries such as The Netherlands, initiatives in relation to the former are evident but there are very few in relation to the latter, while in other countries such as Sweden, the opposite is the case. However, in most countries surveyed by Watters neither group was being catered for adequately or in a systematic way. Yet, as I have stated earlier, the challenges in terms of providing services for refugees and asylum seekers are not substantially different to those in relation to settled minorities; refugees and asylum seekers *are* essentially ethnic minorities.

Struggle within institutional psychiatry

Struggles against racism within professional bodies tend to take diverse forms. Aggressive direct action is often unproductive and difficult, mainly because of the power held by these bodies over its members. The author is aware of some of the ways in which these struggles have shaped up over the years in Britain, especially those struggles with and within the body that represents psychiatrists within the UK, the Royal College of Psychiatrists. The following section provides an abbreviated but personal, and hence limited, view of events over the past twenty years.

For many years psychiatrists and others interested in issues around racism and cultural diversity tended to gravitate towards the Transcultural Psychiatry Society (UK), a multidisciplinary body that came into being following the first International Congress on Transcultural Psychiatry held in Bradford in 1976 (Fernando 1988). Originally, this society, which has become known as the TCPS, was dominated by white psychiatrists who had worked in Asia or Africa, such as Philip Rack and John Cox. Over the next few years the society attracted black and Asian professionals and broadened its interests from academic 'cultural psychiatry' that focused on 'cultural differences' to actual service provision as experienced by patients caught up in what soon became recognised (within the TCPS) as a racist and culturally insensitive mental health system. In April 1985, soon after Aggrey Burke, the first black consultant psychiatrist in the UK, became its president, the constitution of the TCPS was changed to specify the following:

> The objects of the Society shall be the promotion of mental health and advancement of psychiatric knowledge for the public benefit irrespective of race class gender culture and in particular (but without in any way limiting the generality of the foregoing) to increase awareness and understanding of the effects of racism sexism and culture on health and illness and to encourage sensitivity to prejudiced attitudes, racist and sexist practices and cultural values among practitioners who are concerned with mental health.
>
> (1988: xiii)

All through the late 1980s and early 1990s, psychiatrists who were prominent members of the TCPS resisted the idea of forming a 'section' within the Royal College of Psychiatrists (henceforth referred to as the College) although this may have been easily achieved at that time. It was felt (within the TCPS) that such a section would not be given an adequate voice in the College if it highlighted issues that mattered to black people while its very existence (including people prominent in the struggle against racism) within the College would validate the College's general stance in denying racism in psychiatry. In fact at least one of the most prominent members of the TCPS, Sashi Sashidharan, actually resigned from the Royal College of Psychiatrists in protest against (what he saw as) its pro-racist ethos, highlighted by its failure to discipline one of its members who was found to be overtly racist at an appointments committee in 1984 (see Anwar and Ali 1987). However, attitudes changed gradually within the College over the years. In 1990, at the behest of the then Dean of the College (no other than Professor John Cox, one of the founder members of the TCPS), Dr Parimala Moodley, who had been Chairman of the TCPS, led several other psychiatrists (including me) into forming the 'Transcultural Special Interest Group' (TSIG) within the College.

Significantly, the first meeting of the TSIG was devoted almost entirely to voicing resentment by black (mainly Asian) psychiatrists about the discrimination that they faced in pursuing their careers.

The then President of the College reprimanded the TSIG for allowing its first meeting to be used for issues around employment when (as the president saw it) the aim of an interest group was 'academic'. Since then the TSIG has limited its scope to discussing the training of psychiatrists and service provision. The problems of racism in the employment field (faced by its members) has so far been largely ignored by the TSIG, although many within its membership are all too aware of the difficulties faced by black professionals making their way up the professional ladders. In fact it has been left to other people to take this matter up, for example Naz Coker (2001) in a book published recently based on research conducted by the King's Fund. It is significant that the TSIG has attracted little support in terms of active participation by black and Asian psychiatrists although it has a very large nominal membership list. The College frequently marginalizes the TSIG, for example by not providing a prominent platform for its presentations at College meetings, and the TSIG is still to achieve the status of a 'faculty' of the College. A lesson to be learned from the experience of the TSIG is that the preoccupation with their own personal struggles with racism may well be leading black psychiatrists to disregard, or at least avoid confronting, the racism that affects the black people they meet as patients. Books on the general theme of transcultural psychiatry written by some psychiatrists from centres of excellence (*sic*) such as the Institute of Psychiatry, have pursued issues around cultural difference rather than racist oppression. As black psychiatrists are taken on by the psychiatric establishment some tend to get 'taken in', i.e. they become apologists for the College's (and their own institutions') failures, becoming, in the words of Fanon (1967), '"reliable men" [and women] to execute certain gestures' (1967: 34) rather than activists for change. Some of the issues involved are considered further later on in this chapter when the nature of the black response in the mental health field is discussed.

In mid-2001, led by the then President of the College, John Cox, three actions were taken by the College Council (the governing body of the College). First, an 'Ethnic Issues Project Group' was formed leading on to the formation of a 'Special Committee on Ethnic Issues'; second, an external consultancy was brought in to work with the College to examine College structures for institutional racism and to suggest remedies for any deficiencies in this field discovered during this process; and third, proposals were submitted to the College Council aimed at bringing 'transcultural psychiatry' into the curriculum for training psychiatrists (see Cox 2001). The moves made by the College in 2001 are a noteworthy achievement. However, I have some concerns about subsequent developments. The 'Special Committee on Ethnic Issues' was formed in a way that indicated impending tokenism in that members of the College who were knowledgeable and critical about the workings of the College were actively excluded from the committee. Further, a group brought together earlier by the President of the College consisting of black users and their supporters – a group that was supposed to feed into this committee – was in effect disbanded by the College. The indications at the end of 2002 were that the positive moves made earlier by the College were being undermined by the very institutional processes that the moves were supposed to deal with.

Psychiatric training

The training of psychiatrists is overseen by the Royal College of Psychiatrists. In 1995, the TSIG of the College put up proposals to the College Council through the Dean outlining ways in which training should be changed. This group suggested that (a) subjects basic to psychiatry should include the psychologies from Asia and Africa, Asian and African healing, the history of race and racism in psychiatry and psychology; (b) clinical skills training should cover cultural sensitivity; and (c) ethical considerations should address racism in professional practice. The Governing Council of the College shelved discussion of this topic and the document went the rounds of committees for some years until it apparently died.

Following the decision by the College that 'transcultural psychiatry' should be brought into the curriculum for training (see above), a two-day workshop of invited members was held in early February 2001 (Moodley 2002) when 'the knowledge, skills and attitudes of a well-trained and culturally competent psychiatrist' (2002: 63) were agreed and a way forward for changes in training of psychiatrists suggested. Although these meetings were stimulating to attend, my feeling at the end was not very hopeful. Institutional racism was acknowledged as a problem to be faced, but there was no agreement on how this may be done. The responsibility for making changes was left to the Dean of the College. The concept of 'cultural competence' seemed to carry the day implying that racism was best left unstated. In my view, it is very unlikely that any changes in the training of psychiatrists that result from the processes put into effect in 2001–2002 would be anything more than cosmetic ones and they are extremely unlikely to result in *practical* improvements felt by black service users – unless the black members of the College who have achieved some small degree of power within the college (mainly as examiners) take a stand and pursue the issues more vigorously than they have so far done.

Initiatives in mental health service provision

A number of initiatives to deal with the problems experienced by black and Asian people when they confront or access mental health services have come and gone over the past twenty years. There have been ventures, usually transitory, that have attempted to address some of the problems arising from 'ethnic issues' (Chapter 2) within the statutory sector, but no clear indication of a consistent pattern of change. The more important developments that have led to long-term change were initiatives involving community provision of residential facilities often through housing associations, self-help vocational schemes and recreational centres. Mental health workers became involved in some of these, for example the Harambee Housing Project in Birmingham. More recently most of the community projects in the mental health field (usually within the black voluntary sector) have taken the form of psychotherapeutic or counselling services for black and/or Asian people, sometimes with day care. However, some voluntary groups have remained as pressure groups or groups that provided 'expertise' to the statutory sector. Generally most black and Asian groups have been dependent on the commitment of a few people and so none have achieved great prominence in the mental health field. This section is by no means a comprehensive account of initiatives that have tried to address ethnic issues. The projects that I describe here are purely a sample and, in the case of the wholly statutory sector ones, are projects that have been reported on in one form or other.

Statutory sector projects

In this section I refer to four projects, namely the Transcultural Unit in Bradford, the Maudsley Outreach Service Team (MOST) in London, the Home Treatment Service in Birmingham, and 'Ipamo', a project in south London developed as a partnership between the statutory and voluntary sectors. None of these discussions is comprehensive and the views presented are personal ones. Some voluntary sector projects are discussed in the next section headed 'black voluntary sector'. Issues underlying the demise of Ipamo will be addressed later when problems of the black voluntary sector are considered.

In the late 1970s and early 1980s, some statutory bodies (health authorities) promoted the formation of groups of people to 'specialise' in providing services for minority ethnic communities in their areas, usually by employing professionals who were conversant with minority languages and/or minority cultures. One such venture led to the formation of the Transcultural Unit at Lynfield Mount Hospital, Bradford in the early 1980s (see Rack 1982). This was the first attempt in the statutory sector to have a service that set out to address ethnic issues in practical terms. As such it was both innovative and significant. The unit began when Dr Phillip Rack, a white psychiatrist who had developed a special interest in 'transcultural psychiatry', formed a team of professionals from various cultural backgrounds in order to provide a linguistically and culturally sensitive service for Asian people in the area, largely people of Pakistani origin. The Bradford approach became well known and after Dr Rack retired others took over its leadership. In effect, the staff attached to this unit acted as 'specialists' providing a cultural consultancy to mental health services in the district, occasionally taking over the care of people or families referred to it. Essentially it depended on members of the team developing cultural knowledge and, more importantly, being committed to adapting traditional European psychiatry to suit the needs of their clients. The unit thrived for several years but then, about 1988 or so, it appeared to lose support from the hospital organisation and questions were raised about its 'special' status. Finally in 1999, the managers of the Trust decided to close the unit on the basis that its work would be absorbed into the general work of the service, i.e. 'mainstreamed'.

During the 1980s it became apparent that black people might be more accepting of home-based psychiatric services than they were of hospital services, mainly because hospitals had a strong negative image among black people. The results of a survey carried out at the Maudsley Hospital in the 1980s (Moodley 1995) showed that

'While white patients considered the social contacts made through hospital as being more important, African and African-Caribbean patients rated seeing a member of staff of their own colour, being understood and receiving help with finding jobs as more important' (1995: 128). Based on anecdotal reports of similar user views, a new community-based service, the Maudsley Outreach Service Team (MOST) set up in the early 1980s, pursued a user-centred approach. Dr Moodley, a psychiatrist of black South African background who was the director of MOST, writes 'We believe that our success was a result of working *with*, rather than for or at, our patients. Our interventions were always made explicit and nearly always agreed upon between the professionals and service users involved – with compromises on both sides' (1995: 138). In 1990, MOST was 'mainstreamed' by the Maudsley Hospital. This meant that its functions were placed within the main mental health service structure of this hospital. What happened in effect was that its activities were disbanded.

Another significant development, built on an emphasis on home-based services, is the North Birmingham Home Treatment service under the direction of Professor Sashidharan that started as the West Birmingham Home Treatment Service (Parveen 1995). This service began in 1990 when a ward at All Saints Hospital was closed allowing resources dedicated to that ward to be transferred into community work in the area previously served by that ward. This arrangement was initially a pilot project serving a population of 35,000. Later, when it was shown to be successful, the scheme was widened to serve a catchment area of 200,000 forming part of the services provided by the North Birmingham Mental Health Trust. Over sixty per cent of the clients dealt with by the service are from ethnic minority backgrounds. The staff are said to be committed to 'anti-oppression practice' (1995: 9) and are mainly black people themselves. They claim that black clients find the service particularly acceptable because it employs mainly black staff and an emphasis is placed on keeping people out of hospital. More recently, specific community-based services have been set up in north Birmingham directed at meeting the mental health needs of black African-Caribbean people and Asian people, these services are the Frantz Fanon Centre and the Asian Resource Centre.

In the early 1990s several black activists interested in mental health issues, primarily Yvonne Christie, developed the Sanctuary Project (Jennings 1996). This was aimed at developing appropriate alternatives to psychiatric hospital care, run by black people for black people. Working groups were formed to develop a project in Hackney (north London) and one in Lambeth (south London), both areas with relatively high black populations. Initially both groups envisaged 'partnerships' between statutory and voluntary sectors. The project for Hackney gradually changed into a voluntary-sector project within a housing association contracting with the local social services department. It now functions as The Nile Centre (see pp. 77–8). The group for Lambeth pursued the partnership pathway hoping to develop a project that would be within the statutory mental health service for the area, eventually funded by the National Health Service once priming funding was discontinued. The project became know as Ipamo. This project will be described briefly below. The lessons that can be learned about problems for partnerships between black agencies and white institutions are discussed later in this chapter under the heading 'Problems of the black voluntary sector'.

Having obtained special funding from the Department of Health, Ipamo was set up in mid-1995 as a voluntary organisation that planned to work in partnership with the statutory bodies that provided the local mental health services for Lambeth (that included Brixton). The arrangement was that the former held responsibility for the funds and capital development while Ipamo, through its Board of Directors, was responsible for the service to be developed. Ipamo developed a service model and a detailed structure for an innovative service to be staffed by black people. The ethos of the service was worked out in meetings and conferences sponsored by Ipamo, and its Board of Directors approved working practices devised by Ipamo's Director Malcolm Phillips, an accomplished mental health professional who was well respected in black communities. The vision for Ipamo was a model of care that brought into traditional approaches to mental health, ideas from black social and political movements combined with notions of spirituality (see Chapter 3). Negotiations with the statutory bodies in charge of the funds were often fraught. Also, Ipamo sensed opposition from psychiatrists and other professional staff although this was not openly expressed. A building was purchased as the location for Ipamo but the statutory bodies concerned (a health authority and a mental health trust) informed Ipamo of various practical problems, such as dismissal of the architects employed for redesigning the building, and a gradual diminution of funds available for service provision. Finally, after about three years of planning and negotiation between Ipamo and the statutory bodies, the latter decided that the project was not viable and stopped funding Ipamo in December 1998. The issues around this misadventure in partnership are discussed further in the section on problems of the black voluntary sector.

Voluntary sector projects

There are numerous mental health projects in the black voluntary sector. Some of these are listed in *Not Just Black and White* (Harding 1995) a book that could do with updating. They face numerous problems (see below) not least the instability of funding, since most are on short-term funding, and the constant struggle against pressures to prove their 'worth', something that few white projects are asked to do with the same sort of insistence. I have seen this from the inside. This pressure is seldom about quality but more to do with satisfying an expectation that they would function 'as expected' (by the statutory services). In other words, although funders pay lip service to 'innovation' in service provision, what they often demand is that traditional types of service provision are given a 'black face'. Also, many funders do not seem to ask for quality checks in terms of responses from (black) users of services, and seem to need assurance that important people (be they councillors or local psychiatrists) support the work. At a more subtle level, what happens quite often is that projects that appear critical of the establishment by following ways of working that are very different to those of the statutory sector get pressurised to produce 'evidence' of their worth, while those that keep a non-critical profile get away with providing very poor accounts of their credibility in the eyes of their clients. Another issue that seems to matter is the ethnic composition of the trustees. I have noted that black projects that do not have white trustees are hard put to prove their worth, while black projects that have few or no black trustees have very little difficulty in this respect.

In this section I shall describe very briefly three projects in the black voluntary sector, having chosen them mainly because I have known them personally at first hand. These are Nafsiyat, which calls itself an Intercultural Therapy Centre, providing counselling and psychotherapy for ethnic minorities in north London, The Qalb Centre, a counselling centre for Asian people in east London, and The Nile Centre, based in Hackney (a London Borough), to provide supported residential facilities, outreach crisis intervention and counselling for black African and African-Caribbean people.

Nafsiyat, set up in 1983, is probably the first centre specifically aimed at providing psychotherapy for ethnic minorities to be set up in the UK. It was founded by Jafar Kareem, a clinical psychologist from Bengal (India) who had been trained in Europe and had been working for some years in the National Health Service. Some of the ideas promoted and developed at Nafsiyat are written up in chapters by Kareem in the book *Intercultural Therapy* (Kareem and Littlewood 2000). The approach at Nafsiyat, when it started, was to emphasise the need to move away from a Eurocentric psychoanalytic model by modifying psychodynamic psychotherapy. I well remember Jafar Kareem saying that if therapy did not suit a client, it was the therapist who had to change and not the client. So his approach was to learn from the black and Asian clients seen at Nafsiyat in order to develop a form of psychotherapy appropriate to them. Jafar Kareem personally supervised all the therapists at the centre and encouraged them to develop a Nafsiyat style of intercultural therapy. Tragically, Jafar Kareem died suddenly in 1992. The 'Nafsiyat style' was an innovation that was very personal to Jafar Kareem and possibly died with him. In fact for about one year before he died, he and I were involved in discussions on developing a centre for people with the sort of problems that led to mental hospitalisation; but it was not to be. The lack of anyone who could provide leadership to Nafsiyat once Jafar Kareem died, and serious internal problems of management between 1997 and 1999, led to Nafsiyat becoming, in my view, a fairly traditional 'white' psychoanalytic psychotherapy centre. Perhaps a few of the therapists still attempt to carry on Jafar Kareem's style of working but my impression is that the centre delivers traditional psychoanalytic psychotherapy within a narrow western tradition.

The importance of Nafsiyat lies in it being the first centre to try and modify western psychotherapy into becoming a mode of therapy that addresses racism and cultural diversity, and hence 'multicultural' in nature. The failure of Nafsiyat to have built on Jafar Kareem's work carries lessons that I pursue in Chapter 5 when I discuss ways in which counselling and psychotherapy could change to address the needs of a multicultural society. Fortunately, many other counselling and psychotherapy services have come on the scene and they may well take things forward in this field.

The Qalb Centre was set up in east London (Waltham Forest District) in 1993 by a group of mainly Asian professionals, including social workers, counsellors and a psychiatrist. The centre aims to provide a holistic form of counselling and complementary therapies for Asian people experiencing mental health problems (Gorman 1995). The complementary therapies available include reflexology, massage and yoga. The counsellors are mainly Asian and they have developed ways of liasing with the complementary therapists in order to complement each other. Therapy provided at Qalb is greatly appreciated by users of the service. More recently, Qalb has set up a day-care centre for Asian people with long-term mental health problems where a 'holistic' approach is being used in the counselling. Most of the clients attending the day-care centre are people referred to Qalb by the statutory psychiatric services. Each client has a programme drawn up which does not take psychiatric diagnosis into account at all, but is based on enhancing the positive aspects of the client's life situation, skills and community support.

The Nile Centre opened in July 1997 as a mental health facility for African and African-Caribbean people within Kush, a black-led housing association. It is funded by grants from various sources, mainly the (statutory) social services department. The Nile Centre offers help during crises with supportive housing, outreach crisis support and counselling. All the staff are of African or African-Caribbean origin and the clients are either self-referred or referred by professionals working in the statutory mental health service in Hackney (a borough in east London). Nearly all the clients have a psychiatric diagnosis attached to them usually indicating 'serious mental illness' but diagnosis is not taken as indicative of the type of intervention offered by Nile. Its ethos is overtly to address the effects of racism, social deprivation and social exclusion, all in a culturally sensitive and 'holistic' framework. This is seen as complementing the medical-model approach of the statutory sector. The staff attempt to liase closely with statutory sector workers who are nearly always involved with the clients of Nile, although their involvement is usually reduced once Nile staff are involved. The approach is to maintain communication between the workers in the two agencies at a grass-roots level, although the project itself is entirely independent of the statutory sector. The results of the work of The Nile Centre has not been critically analysed but anecdotal reports and evaluations of the work carried out by independent bodies suggest that the services are greatly appreciated by its black users.

Problems of the black voluntary sector

The difficulties encountered by the black voluntary sector in general (not just the social care and mental health scene) have been reviewed as far as African-Caribbean projects are concerned in a study by the African-Caribbean Community Development Unit written up by Wenham (1995). I have drawn partly from Wenham's report, *Funded to Fail: Nuff Pain No Gain* (Wenham 1995), to identify some of the problems that have been, and still are, of concern with regard to the mental health field.

General issues

The main problems of the black voluntary sector, as I see them, are charted in Box 2.2. They are mainly based on personal experience and discussion with people working in the voluntary sector.

The first issue is around vulnerability. Many services in the black voluntary sector are dependent on funding from local authorities. What I have noted is that when local authorities look for ways of cutting expenditure, black voluntary groups are easy targets. Usually they lack powerful allies and seem to be struggling along on their own without many connections with other organisations. In some areas, there appears to have been a decline in influential black staff within the local statutory sector who may have supported the groups initially. Quite often black politicians (from whom these groups may expect support) find it difficult to give time for what are relatively small issues for them without many votes. Sometimes what happens is that, in a situation where managers and commissioners feel that they have to show that black projects are being funded, projects that are only nominally 'black' get supported, and these are projects dominated by white management committees with orientations and policies that conform to the expectations of the 'white establishment'.

The second issue concerns support and organisation. Unlike many 'white' projects that are well supported (often sometimes by national organisations such as Mind or Age Concern) and with

Box 2.2 Black voluntary sector weaknesses

Easy target for cuts
   lack of powerful allies
   lack of network support
   small size
   little influence

Inherent structural problems ('funded to fail')
   under-funding
   lack of infrastructural support
   unfair demands by funders
   communication with 'white' establishment

Lack of strategic objectives
   poor community links
   inadequate quality measures
   limited user involvement in management

structures firmly founded as a result of many years of functioning, many black voluntary groups have structural problems and very little support from national organisations. Often they have little infrastructural support and depend very much on the commitment of one or two people. Even when a local authority provides some sort of support this is usually through a support service that itself is under-funded and sometimes closely tied up with other large voluntary organisations (the general or white voluntary sector) in the area. Management committees drawn from black communities often seem ill equipped to take on the sort of complex issues presented to them in the face of very heavy demands being made by funders, often much heavier that those made on other voluntary groups. Often there are clear double standards being applied. No doubt stereotypes and cultural communication problems play some part in this too. Finally, the funding given is often inadequate for the purpose and linked to unreasonable expectations.

   Thirdly, many black groups lack clear strategic objectives and just run out of steam. This can happen when a project that began as a result of the energies and vision of one or two people, loses the founders for whatever reason, without the project being bound up with the community it claims to serve. Then, what could happen – and does happen sometimes with the connivance of statutory funders – is that the project becomes a mere copy of the statutory sector provision, possibly living on an established reputation merely paying lip service to being a 'black service'; in other words it becomes to all intents and purposes a part of the statutory sector, albeit run by black or Asian people. This raises issues of internalised racism and the way power gets exercised, and about tokenism.

In the mental health field the advantages of successful ethnic-specific projects are obvious. They are relatively free to innovate and culturally interpret the concepts of counselling and psychotherapy, not being hedged into clear-cut styles of working and theories as are services based on traditional psychiatry and psychology. These ethnic-specific projects generally attract people with ideas and imagination, who, although trained as counsellors or psychotherapists, can and do adapt traditional western systems or even bring into counselling new ways of thinking and working, and anti-racist dimensions. From a cultural standpoint too, most of the counsellors and psychotherapists in the black voluntary sector claim that they do not work in a eurocentric way and that they have moved away from what they were taught in their training. How exactly this works out must vary a great deal but this does say something about the training available at present in the UK. This point is explored further in Chapter 5.

Many mental health projects in the black voluntary sector are clearly very popular with users of the service, but they have inherent problems as well as the ones described earlier (pp. 78–80). As far as I can see, nearly all these projects find it difficult to build up their therapeutic skills, partly because of the instability of being on short-term funding and sometimes also because they lack in-built quality measures and accountability to the communities they serve. To assume that because a project has a black manager and black therapists they are in tune with the needs of black clients can be very misleading. Another problem is that there are no clear models of counselling for such centres to follow and so they have to each invent the wheel for themselves or fall back on almost unwittingly following what is referred to as 'eurocentric' models.

Voluntary–statutory partnership

Partnership between the voluntary and statutory sectors seems, on the face of it, one way of getting round some of the problems outlined above. However, there are I believe particular difficulties when black voluntary groups become involved too closely with the statutory sector. The story of Ipamo exemplifies some of these.

Ipamo was a well-funded ambitious project hailed at the time it was inaugurated as a model for an ethnic-specific service for African-Caribbean people. In the end it failed miserably with recrimination all round, the health bodies blaming the black people who planned the project and the latter blaming the health bodies for mismanaging the finances and the capital development. The people who lost were the black communities of Lambeth. The truth is difficult to define but, since I was a member at one time of its Board of Management, I can claim to have some knowledge from which lessons can be drawn.

The partnership between Ipamo and the Health Trust for the district concerned was started in mid-1995. What happened in practical terms was that joint working between Ipamo and the Trust broke down over the next three years, or perhaps it was an association that never really developed into a firm partnership. The arrangement was that the funds allocated by the Department of Health were given to the local Health Authority to be administered by the Health Trust of the area served by Ipamo. The Trust was responsible for the capital development and for meeting the resource needs of Ipamo as it developed services. There were various delays in the capital development. On numerous occasions, the Trust told Ipamo that money allocated for services would be required to meet shortfalls in capital needs because of various 'problems', the real nature of which were never clear. What Ipamo saw was the gradual eroding of the money that Ipamo could claim for services through what was perceived as mismanagement by the Trust. But when challenged, the Trust blamed Ipamo for giving bad advice and misusing funds, quoting a relatively small amount spent on a conference arranged with the full approval of the Trust. Finally, after the money available had dropped by one third, the Trust and Health Authority stated that the whole project would need rethinking and disbanded Ipamo.

In my opinion, the primary fault was that the two sides of the 'partnership' did not negotiate with all their cards on the table. Ipamo was committed to a certain vision and suspected that the other side would try to undermine it, so at Ipamo we kept our cards close to our chest. The statutory bodies did not question the vision but avoided participating in discussing it. The only opposition to the vision came from vague comments made by consultant psychiatrists of the Trust casting doubt on the feasibility of implementing the vision proposed by Ipamo. Clearly these misgivings would have been relayed to the Trust managers. What now seems (to me) to have been a fundamental dispute was never openly addressed or even properly verbalised. Secondly, the power differential between the health bodies and Ipamo was not openly acknowledged as a possible source of conflict. The fact that all the members of Ipamo's management committee were black people and all the managers at senior level at the Trust were white was something never commented upon by either side, until after the breakdown had occurred and it was then too late to discuss the possible problems that were inherent in that situation. Also, underlying 'racial' feelings were perhaps never acknowledged. Everyone voiced commitment to a black project but what this actually meant in practice was never spelled out. If tensions had been voiced early on, some way may have been found to build a joint working partnership; perhaps through strategies such as including white people on the Ipamo management committee and black people brought in on their side by the Trust.

The main lesson from the Ipamo fiasco is that a partnership between a powerful white institution and a relatively weak black organisation could be fraught. In fact, such partnerships could even lead to re-enactment of colonial arrangements, where a powerful and prestigious white institution abstracts resources from a weak black organisation, especially since it is easy for prestigious organisations to corrupt staff into colluding in such arrangements, sometimes by offering personal advantages to individuals. I am personally aware of such a situation. In this instance a voluntary organisation that was funded to provide a service for minority ethnic communities became closely associated with a university department in running a course approved by the university for a degree. This course was presented to both students and to the board of directors of the voluntary body as being jointly organised between that body and the university department. What had actually happened was that the black director of the voluntary organisation had been given an honorary post by the university, and facilities and staff time of the voluntary body were devoted to the course. The crunch was that all the fees paid by the students, and these were not inconsiderable, were pocketed by the university. In effect, resources given to the voluntary body by its funders for the benefit of black clients were used to subsidise the course to the financial gain of the university. When called on to explain, the university authorities took the line that the black voluntary organisation obtained hidden benefit from being associated with a prestigious university. The white institution took the money and the black clients suffered.

Black response within mental health

The realisation of the extent and nature of some of the racial and cultural issues that statistics pointed to (Chapter 1), together with some occurrences, such as the deaths in forensic hospitals of black youngsters, led to deep concern and anger among black people generally. Gradually, constructive strategies were formulated, especially as black professionals began to voice their concerns from within the professions of social work and psychiatry, and later even psychology. What seemed to develop sometimes were uneasy alliances between black people located within 'white systems' that were racist in one way or other, and black people outside these systems. The issues of tokenism by the establishment was seen as a problem because some of the black professionals did not seem to join the struggle that gradually developed, at least did not do so openly. There was a feeling among people outside these institutions, and among some black people within them who were involved in struggling against racism, that these 'tokenistic' black professionals were obstructing change. However, at the same time there was appreciation of the difficulties faced by black people working in white institutions.

A significant change over the past twenty years has been the increase in the numbers of black people achieving positions of some influence as professionals in the field of psychiatry, and less so in psychology. Clearly, having black and Asian people in higher echelons of the professions or in positions of some prominence is very important for various reasons, not least because they are in a good position to understand and even counteract the effects of racism in service provision. Although this is welcome, for complex reasons this very fact sometimes hinders progress. Too often, token appointments are quoted as achievements without any assessment of performance at the level of service delivery and this applies to some voluntary sector projects as well as to some statutory services. Another factor in the slowing down of change towards redressing racial inequalities in mental health services, or even the worsening of inequalities that occurred in the early 1990s, was that some (middle-class) black and Asian professionals allowed their presence to be used as a reason for not pursuing change; not usually because they wished to identify as 'honorary white people' but by settling for accepting a racialised discourse so long as they were able to pursue their individual successes in career development and/or material gain, using their blackness to buy into white institutions without making any effort to change them also. In my view, effecting change (of white institutions) 'from the inside' is a necessary approach and one that black and Asian people must continue to pursue. However, the difficulties of being involved are not something to be taken lightly. Explorations of my own experience in this field as a member of the Mental Health Act Commission is briefly described earlier in this chapter and also in a journal paper (Fernando 1996). The conclusions of that paper state that

> black people who wish to fight racism must become involved in British institutions, pushing their way forward if necessary, but once they are involved, they must (in order of priority): (a) be constantly vigilant and not mistake words for actions; (b) push the frontiers of anti-racism as far as possible, making alliances with anyone who wishes to co-operate; and (c) be prepared to confront racism thoughtfully and realistically.
>
> (1996: 152)

Black psychiatrists

An important trap that black and Asian professionals may fall into is the long-recognised one of unwitting, or semi-unwitting, collusion with racism. The involvement of black people in condoning, and hence validating, institutional racism should not surprise anyone who has read Fanon, for example *Black Skin, White Masks* (Fanon 1952) or Fanon's later paper 'Racism and Culture' included in the book *Toward the African Revolution* (Fanon 1967). After all, the British empire was largely run by a black middle class, black slaves were held down by other black slaves, and Jews were used to round up other Jews for transportation to gas chambers. But political liberation movements in Asia and Africa too were led by black people – often middle-class black people. And as Walvin (1993) points out, slavery in British possessions was always 'marked by black resistance' (1993: 278).

The position of black psychiatrists, like many other black professionals, is complicated by the fact that they work in an essentially racist system. Progress up the career ladder often depends on the degree to which individuals collude with or deny racism both in their employment arrangements and in established ways of working. Being too upfront about racism of any sort, even that masked by euphemisms such as 'cultural issues', is not encouraged (and is counterproductive in career progress) while (psychological) denial or (practical) silence is looked upon favourably. Hence, many professionals who achieve positions of some influence are those who are adept at collusion with, and/or denial of, racism sometimes as a strategy but sometimes through blindness.

In my view, most black psychiatrists in the UK appreciate the fact of racism in mental health services and are aware of the racist injustices faced by black users of the services. But many do not see any way in which their actions – or even their speaking out – can alleviate this state of affairs. Their attitude is to keep their heads down and get on with their jobs, helping individually whenever they can but usually taking care not to rock the boat of the psychiatric establishment. Others have so internalised the culture of psychiatry, including its racist aspects, that they fail to see any problem. In fact, I am aware of some black (and Asian) psychiatrists who have much less understanding of racism in psychiatry than do many of their white colleagues. However, there are a few 'rotten apples' who appear to take up collusion actively and deliberately, thereby giving respectability to institutional racism in the places they work, while using their 'black' credentials to pursue career advancement in specialisms such as 'cultural psychiatry' – black skins, white masks with a vengeance. Yet there are several black psychiatrists who also pursue these specialisms but still continue to further the anti-racist cause in one way of the other, for example by researching race topics in a novel way, writing critical articles and speaking out.

Summary

The struggles against racism in society at large have been replicated in the mental health field. Both generally, and in the mental health field, the responses to racism have been varied and often uncoordinated. Following the publication of the Macpherson Report in 1999, government policy underwent a dramatic change for the better in its approach towards countering racism. But the

American–British 'war against terrorism' appears to have set the clock back many years in this respect. The official response to inequities arising from cultural diversity and racism within mental health services is exemplified by the way the Royal College of Psychiatrists has moved from denial through avoidance to half-hearted plans to institute changes in the training of psychiatrists. But the main response has been in highlighting the details of the inequities and developing services that aim to counteract the causes of the inequities – especially ethnic-specific services in the black voluntary sector. Yet the black voluntary sector faces major problems. The position of black and Asian people working within essentially racist systems is fraught; this is reflected in the varied nature of the 'black response' to racism, including the variety of ways in which black and Asian psychiatrists have dealt with the situations they find themselves in.

Part II

Underlying themes

Chapter 3

Psychiatry and mental health from a transcultural perspective

In all societies religious healing and methods of liberating the individual from troubles of the mind tend to exist side by side with naturalistic treatment of ailments with medicines, surgery and physical manipulations, but their sphere of influence tends to shrink in the face of secularisation and scientific medicine (Frank 1963). As western secular constructions of the mind separated out from previously 'religious' understandings of human thinking, feeling and behaviour, and the western medical approach to problems associated with the human condition developed in the eighteenth and nineteenth centuries, psychiatry and western psychology arose as specialisms in the western cultural tradition. I refer to *western* psychology because, unlike the case with psychiatry, one can recognise forms of psychology, the study of the mind, in non-western cultural settings too. Looked at in simple terms, the tradition of recognising illnesses or disorders of the mind and providing 'therapy' for them, in other words psychiatry as it is known today, is not evident in medical traditions of Asia, Africa or pre-Columbian America. Similarly, what is referred to as 'psycho-therapy' and 'counselling', i.e. therapies that employ talking as the main or only tool, appear to be specific to a European cultural tradition. But the situation is not as simple as that.

If one looks at the general issue of mental health transculturally and in some depth, comparing and contrasting traditions is complicated and difficult. Complicated because traditions themselves are not clear and differences and similarities between them are intertwined. Difficult because if, for example, we start from a western viewpoint using concepts, categories and the like that we are familiar with and try to find them in settings where these concepts and categories may have little meaning, there are bound to be problems of interpretation; this is the issue of 'category fallacy' (Kleinman 1977: 4) noted in Chapter 1. And when we try to compare and contrast concepts such as 'mental health' or 'illness' in a context where there are underlying assumptions about inferiority and superiority of ideologies and ways of thinking, the problems get compounded. Although 'psychotherapy' and 'mental illness' (as defined in western cultural traditions) are not recognisable as entities in non-western cultural traditions, this does not mean that the latter traditions do not have means of identifying mental health problems or ways of alleviating such problems. What it does mean is that cultural interpretation is needed in a context where cultural arrogance (akin to racism) is counteracted. In other words, when we say or imply, as I do sometimes in this book, that psychiatry is unknown in non-western traditions and psychotherapy is ethnocentric to European cultures, one should not leave it at that but should look more closely at both sides (as it were) allowing as far as possible for differences in ways of thinking about health, illness and treatment.

In his classic book *Shamans, Mystics and Doctors*, Sudhir Kakar (1984), a western trained psychotherapist working in India, observed that non-western cultures have traditions 'concerned with the restoration of what is broadly termed "mental health" in the West' (1984: 3); and he explored these traditions in India by examining and explaining to western readers the nature of services being provided by some indigenous therapists. Traditional Chinese medicine is generally held to be based on physical interventions, the best known being herbal remedies and acupuncture. But we all know that the mind–body dichotomy is significantly absent in the thinking underlying traditional Chinese medicine and so to describe it as being based on physical interventions may be misleading. In his book *Dragon Rises, Red Bird Flies*, Leon Hammer (1990), a psychiatrist and practitioner of Chinese medicine, offers a new way of viewing Chinese medicine from a western standpoint. He suggests, that Chinese medicine is more akin to psychology or psychotherapy in the western idiom than it is to a medical system (in western idiom): 'Chinese medicine, like most psychotherapies, is concerned with an individual's unique physical and emotional state. Chinese medicine and psychology also have systematic classifications of disease; however, the diagnostic and treatment modes of these practices emphasize the distinguishing intrinsic attributes of each individual' (1990: 3).

Thus, both Indian medical traditions and Chinese medicine include ways of intervening that are 'psychological' (in the idiom of western tradition) and I believe that the same conclusion applies to African medical traditions. So we may refer to them as psychologies or psychotherapies if we accept a very broad definition of what they mean, as Kakar (1984) does. However, I think the situation is somewhat different in considering psychiatry, which is a complex system with not just psychological components but also medical, ethical, political and spiritual aspects (see Fernando 2002). While one can refer to different types of psychology (including the psychology of Chinese medicine) the term 'psychiatry' is best limited to the system that has developed in the west.

Science and religion started to become separate disciplines from the sixteenth century onwards as 'science' came to the forefront in the western tradition. Consequently, ideas about spirituality were generally excluded from both psychiatry and western psychology as these disciplines developed 'scientific' approaches. Yet, it may be said that in practice spirituality and religion have never lost their relevance to mental health and concepts of disordered health. So, many people who use mental health services, and indeed some professionals involved in providing these services, seem to feel that a secularised approach (in psychiatry and psychology) is a drawback, rather than an advantage. In Britain, this feeling is particularly evident among black and Asian people. Voices have been raised even within psychiatry calling for the discipline to reconsider the place of religion and spirituality in psychiatry (e.g. Turbot 1996). Over the past two or three decades religious institutions, perhaps with the exception of Islam, have lost most of their influence over people in the UK and North America. So what is understood as 'spirituality' has drifted away from what is referred to as 'religion'; spirituality and religion are no longer identical concepts in the experience of most people. In fact, many people who claim to be spiritual do not necessarily adhere to an established belief system that it promoted by a specific religion.

Medicalisation of madness and distress

In this section, I present the historical background to modern mental health care, tracing how the concept of 'mental illness' developed in a western tradition. Then, as examples of the way illnesses are constructed in the field of mental health, I describe in some detail two concepts commonly used in the psychiatric system as diagnoses of 'illness': schizophrenia and depression.

Although there are reports of enlightened care for 'mad' people in Chinese, Egyptian and Indian civilisations (Rumbaut 1972), it was in the Arabic Empire, that extended in its heyday between the tenth and thirteenth centuries from Persia to Spain, that a specifically medical approach to the care and treatment of 'madness' appears to have first developed. The Islamic medical approach followed the tradition set by Galen in the second century AD, itself based on Hippocratic medicine of ancient Greece. A scheme of classification for psychic disturbances had gradually developed (Dols 1992):

> Primary acute forms of mental disorder that were associated with fever were called phrenitis and lethargy because of their symptoms of excitement and depression respectively, and primary chronic forms without fever, which were called mania and melancholia because the first was generally characterised by excitement and the second by depression.
>
> (1992: 25)

In essence, medical knowledge from Greek and Indian sources was re-worked after being translated into Arabic and, in the course of this, a definitive medical approach to madness emerged in medieval Islamic society.

Descriptions of madness as medical illnesses in the Arabic Empire have been reviewed in a classic book by Dols (1992), *Majnūn: The Madman in Medieval Islamic Society*. The medical encyclopaedia of Ibn Sīnä or Avicenna (d. AD 1037) contained descriptions of many (medical) mental illnesses, such as melancholia (with and without delusions), loss of memory, lethargic sleepiness, phrenitis (mental disturbance with fever), mania (mental disturbance and agitation without fever) and passionate love – 'a delusionary illness similar to melancholia' (1992: 84). As institutions were established for care of the sick and distressed in the Arabic empire, each general hospital, *bīmäristän* or *märistän*, provided special provision for the insane. A *märistän* was established in Cairo (Egypt) in AD 683, in Aleppo (Syria) in AD 755, in Baghdad (Iraq) in the late eighth century AD, in Kayseri (Caesarea) in AD 1205–1206, and in Granada (Spain) in AD 1365–1367, all at a time when Europe was in its 'dark ages'. In the late middle ages (fourteenth and fifteenth centuries), as many of these institutions became primarily concerned with the care of the mentally deranged 'the word *märistän* came to mean an insane asylum' (Dols 1992: 112–13).

Dols (1992) quotes descriptions of how the insane were treated in the *märistäns* of medieval Islamic society. He notes references to beatings and physical restraint, dispensing of medicines, the use of music, decoration to 'cheer the deranged' and 'music played for their benefit' (1992: 121). According to him, the Turks carried on the tradition of supporting such asylums in the Ottoman Empire (that partially replaced the Arabic empire) into the early twentieth century (1992: 117). The first mental hospital in non-Arabic Europe was established in Valencia (Spain) in 1417, possibly as an imitation of a *märistän*, and it still survives (although now housed in a former monastery) as the Psychiatric Hospital of Father Jofré (Rumbaut 1972). However, the era of the 'great confinement' (Foucault 1967: 38) in Europe (when large numbers of people were institutionalised in asylums devoted exclusively to the socially undesirable classified as 'insane') was to come much later in the seventeen and eighteenth centuries. Although the Arabs were the first to develop a comprehensive medical approach to madness and to hospitalise people designated as mad, the social position of the *märistäns* in medieval Islamic society was very different to that of the 'insane asylums' in seventeenth and eighteenth century Europe. The *märistäns* did not function as repositories for 'the "great confinement" of the socially undesirable' (Dols 1992: 129); the numbers of insane people in *märistäns* were small, some patients were neither poor nor disreputable; märistäns were usually located in the centre of a city, accessible to visitors, and 'accepted matter-of-factly' (1992: 128) by society.

The serious medical study of human behaviour that led to modern-day psychiatry emerged in the late sixteenth century when an interest in matters to do with the mind developed in European medical circles and the word *psychologia* came into use (Zilborg 1941). *A Treatise of Melancholy* by Timothy Bright (1586) and *The Anatomy of Melancholy* by Robert Burton (1621) were published in English, drawing on Greek works translated into Latin. According to Bynum (1981), medical psychology or psychological medicine, later called 'psychiatry', developed in west European culture through two movements in thinking. First, certain behavioural patterns and kinds of mental states were attributed to disease

meriting medical interest rather than to such postulates as possession by demons, a state of sin, or wilful criminality. Second, there
appeared the idea of the 'mind' as an expression of brain activity.
All this occurred in a context of ideologies about the human
condition arising from Cartesian duality, giving 'the dogma of the
Ghost in the Machine' (Ryle 1963: 17), and later Newtonian
physics promoting a mechanistic world view of the human being
(Capra 1982). Also, society was seen as 'an atomistic' system with
'its basic building block, the human being' (Capra 1982: 55). The
combination provided 'the basis for the value systems of the
[European] Enlightenment [namely] ideals of individualism,
property rights, free markets and representative government'
(Capra 1982: 56), often referred to as 'European values'.

Today, one can look back to see that these 'European values'
(*sic*) of the Enlightenment (a movement of the sixteenth and
seventeenth centuries), emphasising freedom of the individual, were
born at the very time that slavery of black people by white people
(the Atlantic slave trade) – the antithesis of freedom – was in full
swing. Indeed, according to Eze (1997), who has collected in a
book some of the influential writings on race that the Enlightenment produced, the work of major thinkers of the Enlightenment
(including Hume, Kant and Hegel), reveal that '"reason" and
civilization became almost synonymous with "white" people and
northern Europe, while unreason and savagery were conveniently
located among the non-whites, the "black," the "red," the
"yellow," outside Europe' (1997: 5). African-American writer
Toni Morrison (1993) (following Orlando Patterson 1982) is not
surprised by this apparent paradox: 'The concept of freedom did
not emerge in a vacuum. Nothing highlighted freedom – if it did
not in fact create it – like slavery' (Morrison 1993: 38). In other
words, racism is the key to understanding this apparent contra-
diction in European thinking, just as racism is the key to apparent
contradictions in the mental health field, such as black people's
experience of the supposedly 'caring' psychiatric system as
oppressive (see pp. 1–2 and 20–1).

Modern era

It was against the background outlined above that the asylum
movement, called the 'great confinement' by Foucault (1967: 38),
took place in Europe from about 1660, when various groups of

people who were considered deviant in one way or other were institutionalised. Gradually, medical psychiatrists, originally called 'alienists' and later (in England) 'mad doctors', achieved a position of some power and influence in the asylums. However, Porter (1990) points out that although this 'mass ghettoing' (1990: 119) was public policy in France and Germany, it was not so in England until about the mid-eighteenth century. Until 1713 there was one public 'madhouse' (Bethlam at Moorfields in London) in the whole country, and it was not until 1808 that an Act was passed in England even *enabling* local authorities to establish asylums. At first, explanations for insanity among asylum inmates were eclectic. According to a list compiled in 1810, insanity in people admitted to Bethlam was said to have arisen 'from moral and character defects ("pride"), from emotional difficulties ("troubles"), from organic causes ("fevers"), from head wounds ("fractures of the skull"), from the brain or belly ("drink"), from heredity ("family")' (1990: 34). But as asylums for the mad, under *medical* jurisdiction, moved from being purely custodial institutions to places where 'lunacy' (madness) was studied, systems of medical diagnoses were developed using whatever information could be obtained, including classical descriptions of illness by Hippocrates (Zilborg 1941). Each institution tended to develop its own classification. A Congress of Mental Science held in Paris in August 1889 attempted to develop some uniformity and devised the first agreed (European) classification of mental illness shown in Box 3.1. Significantly, there was then no mention of anything resembling the modern concept 'schizophrenia'.

In 1777 William Cullen coined the term 'neurosis' (López Piñero 1983) to convey the notion that nervous function could be disordered without disturbance of structure. But it was not until the first half of the nineteenth century that the term 'psychosis' came on the scene to refer to psychological, experiential states (Berrios 1987), while neurosis referred, at the time, to disturbances in the central nervous system. But the meanings of these two terms changed during the course of the nineteenth century with 'psychosis' being used to refer specifically to the insanities (madness), which were then classified along various lines, a meaning sustained in the modern classification of mental disorders (see pp. 96–7). The view grew that some psychoses were caused by structural changes in the brain or the result of toxic factors (now called 'organic' psychoses), while others, the 'functional psychoses', lacked 'any demonstrable

Box 3.1 International classification of mental
illnesses 1889

1. Mania
2. Melancholia
3. Periodical insanity
4. Progressive systemic insanity
5. Dementia
6. Organic and senile dementia
7. General paralysis of the insane
8. Insane neurosis
9. Toxic insanity
10. Moral and impulsive insanity
11. Idiocy, etc.

Source: Tuke (1890)

cerebral disturbance' (Healy 1990a: 44). (The difference between 'functional' and 'organic' disorders corresponds roughly to that between 'software' and 'hardware' problems in a computer.)

In the nineteenth century, Germany was the centre of psychiatric thinking and the first chair of psychological medicine was established at Leipzig in 1811 (Hunter and MacAlpine 1963). A general theory of degeneration was put forward by Morel (1852) to account for the apparently rising rates of insanity and criminality (and also to account for the so-called primitiveness of various racial groups). From 1883 onwards, Emil Kraepelin produced classification systems based on observing asylum patients. In the fifth edition of his textbook *Psychiatrie*, Kraepelin (1896) revived an idea put forward by Morel (1852) by designating a new illness, which he called dementia præcox, as the culmination of degeneration in an individual. In the eighth edition published in 1909, Kraepelin developed the concept of two insanities comprising 'the dichotomy of dementia præcox and manic-depressive disorder' (Weber and Engstrom 1997: 375), and the former was renamed 'schizophrenia' by Bleuler (1911). Concepts relating to depression (originally called melancholia) and mania had been described by Hippocrates and are known in non-western cultural contexts (although not necessarily as 'illness') but the construct 'schizophrenia' was something 'new' (see p. 99).

In the 1890s, Janet and Charcot in France popularised the term 'hysteria' as an illness, and in the 1920s Freud developed the notion of hysteria as being linked with anxiety in anxiety hysteria, as distinct from conversion hysteria (in simple terms, the basic disturbance of anxiety converted into physical disability). The concept of melancholia developed into that of depression after Meyer (1905) spoke against the use of the older term (see p. 104) and this concept of depression was given a new impetus by Freud (1917) when he linked it to guilt. Apart from a swing into 'empiricism' in the 1950s and 1960s, when no clear discontinuity was seen either between normality and mental illness or between two mental illnesses, psychiatry has remained 'polarised between "biological" and "psychological" approaches to clinical disorders' (Healy 1990b: 1).

I recall the continuum model for illness being fairly popular in some centres in Britain in the 1960s. And about then, perhaps as a result of the anti-psychiatry movement (see Ingleby 1980; Turkle 1980), it became fashionable to emphasise social factors in the aetiology of mental illness leading to the popularisation of 'social psychiatry'. The approach of 'crisis intervention', where patients were seen with their families in their own home, was pioneered at Napsbury Hospital in St Albans (England) by Scott (1960). 'Therapeutic communities' were established in some mental hospitals; the most famous were those at Dingleton Hospital in Scotland (Jones 1968) and at Claybury Hospital in north east London (Shoenberg 1972). The therapeutic-community approach was based on large group work aimed at opening up communication so that patients could develop skills in relating to others and then live in the wider community. But the emphasis was still on medical, rather than sociological, explanations for problems, and diagnosis of illness ruled supreme. In fact, 'social psychiatry' merely emphasised social factors as contributing to illness rather than causing illness, very different to seeing illness as being socially constructed as described by Scheff (1966).

1970s onwards

Since the 1970s, the model for delivery of mental health services adopted in most parts of the UK has been one based on multi-disciplinary community mental health teams backed by beds for in-patients in small units in district general hospitals, day hospitals and day centres. This general approach is based on a model of mental health care, written up as the so-called Camberwell service model (Wing and Haley 1972). People who develop 'mental illness', especially if they are diagnosed as 'schizophrenic', are seen as suffering an acute illness followed by social handicap. So, acute treatment in hospital is followed by rehabilitation, then resettlement with long-term support for supposedly stable residual handicaps. The 'revolving door' (repeated re-admission) is not avoided, the idea is to slow down the revolutions to a minimum by active rehabilitation and support (Watts and Bennett 1983). This type of 'social psychiatry' emphasises social factors in aetiology and rehabilitation but continues to see illness as being primarily biological in nature. Scull (1977) claims that a community approach of this sort allows people with mental health problems to be integrated within 'normal society' with their neighbours, even where these ties had become strained or broken, the aim of therapy being to enable such people to establish social relationships. It is really a reversal of the ideas of a hundred years ago, or even sixty years ago – which were essentially that 'mentally ill' people needed to be separated from society until they got over their 'mental' problems.

In spite of changes in models of service provision, mental health problems continue to be viewed as essentially medical 'illnesses' although, admittedly, community care allows non-medical models of care to be used in some situations, as far as it can be within a legal framework that assumes a medical model. If the (British) National Service Framework (Department of Health 1999) is implemented, the service provision model of the future may shift from that based on generic community mental health teams to functionally specialised teams providing 'functional' interventions such as crisis intervention, home treatment, assertive outreach and rehabilitation. However, something that cannot be ignored in the UK is the increasing emphasis on forensic psychiatry, likely to be exacerbated if the proposals for a new Mental Health Act (Department of Health 2002) is introduced. One consequence of this is the increase in numbers of 'forensic patients' in large private institutions, not dissimilar to the old-fashioned mental hospitals that have been closed down. In fact, while community care encourages non-medical models of care, the medical model of interventionist 'therapies' aimed at control is being re-enforced in the forensic field, possibly covering over social issues of poverty, homelessness and racism. Another issue that cannot be ignored is that, on both sides of the Atlantic, a biological emphasis is increasingly evident within the psychiatric system. There is a worrying emphasis on biochemical and genetic factors, rather than environmental and social ones, as causing violence, for example in the so-called 'violence initiatives' in the US (Breggin and Breggin 1993). These issues are pursued further in the section 'Comments on mental health services' below.

Schizophrenia

Around the turn of the century, Kraepelin appeared to divide a unitary concept of insanity (accepted as a functional psychosis) into two major illnesses, manic-depression and schizophrenia. Since both mania and depression (as melancholia) had been recognised as 'illness' in the western tradition since Greek times, what Kraepelin *actually* did was to construct a new 'illness' – 'dementia præcox' or 'schizophrenia' (as it was later known), based on observing people who had been incarcerated in asylums. Although Kraepelin (1919) claimed that dementia præcox was an 'extremely old' (1919: 232) disease without providing any evidence for saying so, this contention has been strongly questioned (Torrey 1973; Hare 1988; Gottesman 1991; Fernando 1988). Gottesman (1991) notes that 'no unambiguously schizophrenia character appears in Shakespearean drama, despite the bards skill as a word-painter of other kinds of behavioral deviances' (1991: 5). In searching for descriptions of (western) psychiatric illnesses in ancient Indian texts, Bhugra (1992) finds 'descriptions of objectively observable illnesses such as alcoholism and epilepsy' (1992: 167) but no clear descriptions of the symptoms of (western) schizophrenia such as hallucinations, delusions and thought disorder. So, it is reasonable to conclude that Kraepelinian schizophrenia cannot be identified in descriptions of madness in European literature prior to Kraepelin's presentation, and it has not been recognised in non-European cultural settings (apart from its imposition as a result of western influence). However, it should be acknowledged that delusions and hallucinations might have been considered to be indicative of mental illness by some medieval Islamic physicians according to Youssef and Youssef (1996), although one cannot really decipher anything like 'schizophrenia' (as we know it today) being identified as an illness in medieval Arabic writings on medicine as reviewed by Dols (1992) in his classic study.

Degeneration and 'atavism'

The *new* illness to appear in psychiatric nosology early in the twentieth century, namely schizophrenia, was conceived in a context (in Europe) of rising crime rates and increasing numbers of people incarcerated in asylums, the apparent failure by European society to contain criminality and insanity (Pick 1989). Psychiatric and psychological thinking was, at the time, strongly influenced by two concepts: (a) 'degeneration' as a basis for understanding both lunacy and 'racial' inferiority (as inborn qualities of individuals); and (b) 'atavism' that explained criminality and insanity as reversals to primitive stages of racial evolution (see Morel, 1852; Lombroso 1911; Pick 1989). Pick (1989) believes that the concept of degeneration must be understood primarily within the language of nineteenth-century racist imperialism, the time when colonialism and slavery were feeding the ideology of racism into European culture. The underlying thesis inherent in the concept of degeneration was that social conflict, aggression, insanity and criminality were all signs of individual pathology representing reversal (throwback) to a racially primitive stage of development, either mentally, physically or both. As biological ideas of Lamarck and Darwin became influential, the concept of degeneration, involving race thinking, attempted to explain the other side of what was seen as 'progress'; it represented an 'impossible endeavour to "scientise", objectify and cast off whole underworlds of political and social anxiety' (1989: 10).

Lombroso's doctrine of 'atavism', a reversal to primitive stages of evolution, focused on analysing physical features of animals, social deviants and others. Lombroso (1911) produced tables of photographs pinpointing physical features that identified criminality and insanity. He believed that the white races represented the triumph of the human species 'but inside the triumphant whiteness, there remained a certain blackness' (Pick 1989: 136). Thus, the signs of criminality and madness that Lombroso identified in white people were really features of blackness (inherent in black people). In *White Man and the Coloured Man* (quoted by Pick 1989), Lombroso (1871) gave free expression to his own views of black people:

Only we White people [*Noi soli Bianchi*] have reached the most perfect symmetry of bodily form. . . . Only we [have bestowed]

... the human right to life, respect for old age, women, and the weak. . . . Only we have created true nationalism . . . [and] freedom of thought.

(Pick 1989: 126)

By the late nineteenth century, the ideas of degeneration and Lombroso's criminology had reached the wider public through popular writings (Pick 1989; Weindling 1989) and a type of biology with a strong racist message became part of the public discourse on social reform. Eugenic solutions to psychiatric problems were proposed in Germany in the mid-1880s (Weindling 1989) and the biological control of deviant behaviour impressed Kraepelin so much that he 'accepted that patients with existing mental problems should be advised against marriage' (1989: 86). During the 1890s, Forel (in Germany) began to castrate patients as a means of controlling aggression, even then associated with mental problems. In 1918, Kraepelin set up the German Psychiatric Research Institute in Munich with his pupil, Ernst Rüdin, as the head of its Genealogical Department (Weindling 1989: 336). As Rüdin led its research with money from the American Rockefeller Foundation, the institute's main research thrust was to investigate the genetic patterns of what were assumed to be inherited diseases, including schizophrenia. The Institute stressed its aim of protecting the public from dangerous and burdensome mentally ill people and much of its early work consisted of establishing a data bank of people seen in these terms (Weindling 1989: 384). The end result was the sterilisation campaigns of the 1930s and finally the actual medical killing of people diagnosed by psychiatrists as incurably 'schizophrenic'.

The concept of degeneration really took off in England when, combined with the racist eugenics of Francis Galton 'there was a slide into biological idealism . . . into a conception of degeneration as the imagined subject, cause and force of history' (Pick 1989: 199). From the 1880s through to 1900, psychologists, psychiatrists, anthropologists and lawyers elaborated the language of degeneration and eugenically orientated academics, journalists and doctors were involved in its promotion. The mathematician Karl Pearson (1901), then a professor of London University and a Fellow of the Royal Society, justified the extermination of 'inferior races' as being a way of improving human stock. Indeed, by 1912 the influence of a group centred around Pearson, his journal *Biometrika* and his academic department at University College, London, led to London University hosting the first International Congress of Eugenics, with Lord Darwin as president and Winston Churchill as vice-president (Pick 1989: 199). And so racist ideology became as much a part of British psychiatry as schizophrenia, the two being closely linked in psychiatric thinking.

Speculation about 'race'

In parallel with theories about madness among Europeans, there was considerable speculation in the nineteenth century about the nature of the minds of black people and the universality of madness across racial groups. (This argument continues today in discussions about the 'incidence', rather than the 'diagnosis', of schizophrenia in black people.) Two distinct views were discernible then. First, Daniel Tuke (1858) and Maudsley (1867, 1879) in England, Esquirol (cited by Jarvis 1852) in France, and Rush (cited by Rosen 1968) in the US voiced views similar to Rousseau's mid-eighteenth-century concept of the 'Noble Savage', i.e. that 'savages' who lacked the civilising influence of western culture were free of mental disorder. This idea was expressed most firmly by J. C. Prichard (1835) in his *Treatise on Insanity and Other Disorders Affecting the Mind*: 'In savage countries, I mean among such tribes as the negroes of Africa and the native Americans, insanity is stated by all . . . to be extremely rare' (1835: 349). But, according to Aubrey Lewis (1965) a second, somewhat different stance too was evident in Europe about that time, namely the view that non-Europeans (black people) were mentally degenerate because they lacked western culture. In other words, black people already had the quality of degeneration active in them; blackness was equivalent to criminality and madness. (These ideas reverberate today in arguments over genetic and biological explanations versus environmental explanations for the allegedly high incidence of schizophrenia among black people.)

Although the 'Noble Savage' viewpoint idealised non-European culture in some ways and the notion that black people were 'degenerate' vilified it, both approaches sprang from the same source, a racist perception of people and their cultures. Almost into the twentieth century, Babcock (1895), a psychiatrist from South Carolina, was to use pro-slavery arguments to develop the theme that Africans were inherently incapable of coping with civilised life.

In a paper, '*The Colored Insane*', Babcock juxtaposed the idea that mental disease was 'almost unknown among savage tribes of Africa' with the alleged 'rapid increase of insanity in the negro since emancipation' forecasting 'a constant accumulation of [black] lunatics' in the years to come (1895: 423–7).

In the US, psychiatry had been used, in the nineteenth century, to legitimise slavery; for example epidemiological studies based on the US Census of 1840 (Anon 1851) were quoted in claiming that black people were relatively free of madness in a state of slavery 'but that the black man becomes prey to mental disturbance when he is set free' (Thomas and Sillen 1972: 16). During the 1890s, eugenic concepts gained wide support in the US. Laws against marriages between black and white people were widespread (Rogers 1942) and, in 1896, Connecticut passed legislation regulating marriages (between whites) for eugenic purposes and other states soon followed (Grob 1983). Immigration was blamed for an apparent 'increase in insanity and other forms of degeneracy that threatened the biological well-being of the [white] American people' (1983: 168).

Summary of schizophrenia

During the early part of the twentieth century, racism and eugenics became central to German political thinking as ideas about degeneration became central to thinking about madness and crime. Schizophrenia was seen as a form of degeneration and, to some extent, atavism, in both cases involving European ideas about race – racist ideas. In other words, schizophrenia came from the same stable as eugenics (of psychology) and the Nazi movement (of politics). It was perhaps no coincidence that people diagnosed as 'schizophrenic' were the first victims of sterilisation and extermination on sociopolitical eugenic grounds. The ideologies about race, criminality and stigma are deeply embedded in the diagnosis of schizophrenia.

Depression

It has been claimed that of all psychiatric diagnoses depression is the one that raises most issues of cross-cultural validity (Kleinman and Good 1985; Jhadav and Littlewood 1994). It may be the case that depression has been singled out in this respect by researchers because of its academic interest for anthropological and trans-cultural research, and by clinicians because of its popularity as a diagnosis. If looked at from a black service user's point of view – and indeed from the point of view of black communities in Britain – the use of 'depression' is not anywhere near as worrying as the use of 'schizophrenia' as a diagnosis (see pp. 33 and 154–6).

The concept of depression has a long history in western medicine. It started as 'melancholia', described as an illness by Hippocrates (Jones 1823) as early as the fifth or sixth century BC (Jackson 1986). The Greek physician, Aretaeus of Cappadocia wrote about it as an illness in the second century AD (Adams 1856), and the concept accumulated various meanings and theories as it was elaborated in medieval Islamic medicine (Dols 1992) before emerging in the west in the late middle ages (Jadhav 2000). The concept of melancholia was widened in the sixteenth and seven-teenth centuries to such an extent that 'melancholic' became a popular way of describing people in English literature (Lyons 1971). In the post-Renaissance period melancholia was categorised into somatic and psychological types (Jackson 1986). Melancholia was included as a part of manic-depressive illness by Kraepelin in 1896 (Defendorf 1902). The term depression gradually replaced melancholia in the early part of the twentieth century, perhaps, according to Jackson (1986), after Adolph Meyer (1905) spoke strongly suggesting that the term depression be used 'to designate, in an unassuming way exactly what was meant by the common use of the term melancholia' (1905: 114).

Cross-cultural studies

If we take a pragmatic and practical approach to the issues around diagnosing depression cross-culturally, we can see that something like clinical depression can be recognised in Indian literature (Singh 1975) but not as an illness in, say, Ayurveda (the main Indian system of medicine), although depression, or something akin to this, may be seen as a religious or spiritual experience, or more generally as a 'problem' of the human condition; in other words a mental health problem. Margaret Field (1958) observed that many people who attended an Ashanti shrine in Ghana were identifiable as suffering from psychotic depression and obtained help through religious practices (Field was a government ethnologist in the Gold Coast in the 1930s who later studied medicine and psychiatry to return to Ghana in the 1950s). More generally, Field found that what might be diagnosed from a western psychiatric perspective as 'psychotic depression' was common among Ashanti women but that this was not seen as 'illness' but as the inevitable lot of most women (Kraus 1968). In other words, depression was experienced as an existential issue and not one of 'illness'. Marsella (1978 1980), a psychiatrist, argues from a basis of researching reports of depression in various settings that depression (as conceptualised in psychiatry) is difficult to find in many cultures, giving as examples studies among people in Borneo, Malaysia, First Nations of North America (Native Americans and Native Canadians) and many groups in Africa. Social anthropologist Obeyesekere (1985) hypothesises that in the Sinhala-Buddhist culture (of Sri Lanka) a sense of personal hopelessness (that may be interpreted in western psychiatry as depression) is felt as the essential nature of the world where suffering and sorrow (*dukkha*) are one's natural lot, a state to be overcome (generally using meditation) by under-standing the cause of suffering as attachment, desire and craving. He calls this the 'work of culture' (1985: 134).

Unfortunately, most, perhaps all studies published in psychiatric journals ignore category fallacy (Kleinman 1977) referred to in Chapter 1, and so they are difficult to evaluate. Some fail to avoid obvious racist influences. The first transcultural observation in psychiatry is attributed to Kraepelin (1904) who stated that depression was rare among the Javanese and that guilt was not often seen in Javanese people who became depressed. After that there were several reports of apparent rarity of depression among African-Americans in the US, among Africans (in Africa) and to a lesser extent among Indians in India. Kraepelin (1921) deduced from his observations that the Javanese were 'a *psychically underdeveloped* population' akin to '*immature* European youth' (1921: 171, italics in original). And researchers in Africa and the US attributed the rarity of depression among black people to their 'irresponsible' and 'unthinking' nature (Green 1914: 703) or to an absence of a 'sense of responsibility' (Carothers 1953: 148). Raymond Prince (1968), reviewing twenty-eight reports of depression among Africans between 1895 and 1964, found that a distinct change occurred around 1957 when Ghana became independent. 'In the Colonial era depressions should not be seen and named because Africans were not responsible; in the era of Independence, depressions should be seen because Africans are responsible and aware.' He concluded that 'observing psychiatrists were being influenced in what they were able to diagnose by the prevailing climate of opinion at the time' (1968: 186). In other words, the diagnosis of depression was biased by what we would now call institutional racism.

Before the 1939–1945 war and the Jewish holocaust, depression was reported as particularly prevalent among European Jews compared to non-Jewish Europeans (e.g. May 1922; Strecker and Ebaugh 1931) and a similar picture was reported in the US (e.g. Malzberg 1931, 1962). But this difference was not seen in the new state of Israel (Hes 1960), although rates of depression among Ashkenazi Jewish immigrants were found to be higher than those among Sephardic Jews. Perhaps these observations indicate that depression was related to discrimination or oppression in some way, or to minority status. In general, the 'knowledge' that has emanated from traditional psychiatric studies is that the experience and expression of depression as a somatic (bodily) feeling is much more common among non-western populations and among minority ethnic groups in the west; and that the concept of guilt that emanates from a western Judeo-Christian culture may not be relevant in other cultural contexts. When constellations of emotional distress were given culturally meaningful names they were called 'culture-bound' syndromes (e.g. Lebra 1976; Simons and Hughes 1985); and some of these have been re-interpreted as variants of depression, for example 'soul loss' or 'susto' (Logan 1979) seen in South America, and 'wiitiko' (Parker 1960) among Inuit in the Arctic regions of North America (see Fernando 1988).

I have extracted three approaches to cross-cultural variations that have been proposed by researchers who looked at depression in some depth (Box 3.2).

According to Murphy (1973) a sense of failure rather than guilt is the primary disturbance in depression. This is elaborated by culture depending on how 'self' is differentiated from 'other'. If differentiation is slight this failure is felt as loss of group membership, if stronger it is felt as other people being critical (i.e. shame) and if very strong as failure towards oneself (a sort of 'selfish failure' or guilt). Marsella (1978) suggests that depression becomes recognisable as an entity in cultures that psychologise experience, where the mind–body dichotomy is strong. Obeyesekere (1985) postulates that affects identified as 'depression' in western society are seen as 'illness' because they are 'free-floating' rather than being 'intrinsically locked into larger cultural and

Box 3.2 Cross-cultural variation of 'depression'

Sense of failure or loss is primary disturbance

Experienced in context of differentiation of 'self' vs 'other'
  Loss of group membership ('isolation')
  Failure towards others ('shame')
  Failure towards oneself ('guilt')

Source: Murphy (1973)

Depression occurs in cultures that 'psychologize' experience

Source: Marsella (1978)

Depression is an illness in cultures where 'depressive affects' are free-floating and not tied to issues of 'existence'/religion

Source: Obeyesekere (1985)

philosophical issues of existence and problems of meaning', i.e. 'religion' in a broad sense. So what in some cultures may be thought of as an 'illness' may well be appropriately dealt with by others as a spiritual problem or a way to enlightenment.

Comments on mental health services

When the National Health Service came into being in Britain in 1948 the biological approach to psychiatry of the German–British school dominated the scene. Mental health services and psychiatric services were synonymous. In the US, where psychiatry had been strongly influenced in the 1940s and 1950s by psychoanalytic ideas taken there by European migrants, the approach was less biological and more psychological. The next four decades between 1950 and 1990 saw massive changes in the practice of psychiatry in the UK and in many other parts of the western world. Also over the past twenty or thirty years, especially with the shift from institutional care to community care, there have been changes in the style and content of service delivery reflected in changes in language used. What were once described as 'psychiatric units' are now invariably called mental health services, not even mental disorder services. In these units the term mental illness is being replaced by 'mental health problem', 'psychiatric treatment' by 'mental health interventions' or just 'therapy', and people who were 'patients' are now called 'service users' (except by the die-hard biologically minded psychiatrists). But more importantly, professionals from a variety of backgrounds with a diversity of training are involved in providing these services, usually working as a team. So, while twenty years ago mental health services and psychiatric services were identical, i.e. psychiatry determined almost entirely the models on which mental health services were based, the situation now is somewhat different, at least in developed countries of western Europe and North America. Whether the actual practice of psychiatry or the impact of mental health services on the service user is better or worse than it was fifty years ago is another matter.

Practice of psychiatry

In 1952, chlorpromazine was tried out experimentally for the treatment of mental illness (Delay *et al.* 1952) and by 1954 it was being used clinically (Healy 1990a). Since then many drugs that claim to affect 'mental' functions, i.e. neuroleptics, have appeared and, together with the anti-depressants which first appeared in 1958, have revolutionised psychiatric practice. But together with the advent of widespread use of neuroleptics in the late 1950s and 1960s, many large mental hospitals began to discharge their inmates into the community, the movement of 'de-institutionalisation' (Scull 1977). The result has been a decrease in size of the mental hospital populations in most European countries. The run-down of institutionalisation may well have been a part of the changes in attitude in western Europe after the defeat of fascism, reflected in the development of the welfare state in Britain, de-colonisation and a humanitarian approach to people generally. The part played by the advent of neuroleptics is a matter for debate. In some Scandinavian countries the emptying of mental hospitals had actually started before these drugs were available and the change was attributed there mainly to a change in staff attitudes. Whatever the underlying reasons for the changes, by the early 1960s there was an air of optimism that psychiatry was in the throes of a revolution. Yet, although the policy to close mental hospitals was announced in 1961, large-scale closure of these hospitals did not happen in the UK until the 1980s.

In the US, Thomas Szasz (1962) in *The Myth of Mental Illness* and sociologists such as Thomas Scheff (1966) challenged the traditional biological view of mental illness. In Britain similar views developed into the so-called anti-psychiatry movement led by Laing and Esterson (Cooper 1970), although here illness, particularly schizophrenia, was not denied as an individual reality but was perceived as a way of coping within families – essentially seen as pathological families – as use was made of concepts such as the 'double-bind' (Bateson *et al.* 1956). A residential establishment, Kingsley Hall, was set up in the east end of London in the late 1960s, its work being described vividly in *Two Accounts of a Journey Through Madness* (Barnes and Berke 1971). The Arbours movement with its houses for people with mental health problems is the modern counterpart of the Laingian movement.

Today there is a vast array of neuroleptics – now called 'antipsychotics' – in the *British National Formulary* (Mehta 2002), the standard publication on drugs distributed to all doctors practising in the National Health Service. I recall that even as late as 1959 (when I entered clinical practice after qualifying as a doctor) I was taught that chlorpromazine should be used with great caution and in small doses because of its unknown side effects. Today neuroleptics are used in enormous doses and a multitude of mixtures. The availability of drugs that are overtly promoted as targeting specific illnesses has been the major factor in emphasising the Kraepelinian diagnosis of schizophrenia as a gold standard of good practice. Anti-depressants too have flourished and *pari passu* the diagnosis of depression has soared in popularity over the past two decades. The promotion of drug therapies as therapies for specific illnesses, rather than (as I believe they are) non-specific tranquillisers (see Chapter 5), has resulted in changing attitudes towards what psychiatric illness means, not just among psychiatrists and other professionals but in society at large: 'The knowledge of psychiatry over the last 30 years has been gradually reconstructed by the adoption of neo-Kraepelinian thinking in the USA, which culminated in the hegemony of DSM IV, which classifies mental illnesses in terms of specific diseases' (Donald 2001: 428). In other words, American psychiatry has become Kraepelinian just like the European version. And both have turned increasingly to narrow biological thinking seeing illness as biological entities that have biological remedies, namely drugs.

It is difficult to pin the blame for the shift on to biological thinking, with an emphasis on diagnosis, on psychiatrists and the psychiatric service alone. Public expectations play a large part too. I recall that in my last appointment as a consultant psychiatrist, the one major complaint against the team that I led was that we had not made a diagnosis of schizophrenia early enough and so delayed treatment (i.e. medication). The fact was that our team had been conducting family interviews in the case of a young man referred to us because of alleged angry outbursts towards his parents, being inattentive, refusing to attend the day hospital and running away from home. The parents became increasingly frustrated when the weekly interviews went on for several months and finally left the district with their 'sick' son to stay with relatives in Birmingham. There, the young man was taken to a hospital where a diagnosis of schizophrenia was made after one interview. He was 'stabilised' (i.e. became well behaved) on a fairly high dose of 'anti-psychotic' medication and when the family returned to London an official complaint was made by the parents that the delay in diagnosis had added to the stress that they had faced in caring for a 'mentally ill person'.

Biological hypotheses for schizophrenia and depression, based on the modes of action of the 'anti-psychotic' and 'anti-depressant' drugs appeared in the 1960s and 1970s. Like the number of drugs promoted by pharmaceutical companies as 'cures' for schizophrenia and depression, these hypotheses too have multiplied since then. Although completely unproven in spite of much research, these 'biological' hypotheses remain very much in the forefront of thinking, not just within psychiatry but also within society at large. One reason for this may be that neuroleptics do seem to suppress the feelings and emotional states that are considered to be 'symptoms' of illness because they, the feelings and emotional states, have become medicalised during the two hundred years of psychiatric conditioning of society. However, David Healy (1990a) draws attention to other sociopolitical factors also being important for the ascendancy of biological hypotheses, by comparing the current situation to that in the early twentieth century.

> But other factors seem [to be] suggested by the example of the adoption of morbid heredity and degeneration in French psychiatry precisely 100 years earlier. At this time French psychiatrists were beset by problems. The public held them in low repute. The magistracy derided their claims to legal expertise. The profession was sharply divided along theoretical lines. The situation faced by psychiatry . . . 100 years later.
>
> (1990a: 67)

The reasons for this apparent reversal of psychiatry to the thinking of the late nineteenth and early twentieth centuries will be pursued further in Chapter 5 and Chapter 6.

Emphasis on diagnosis

Clinical psychiatry, at the time of writing, emphasises diagnosis to an extent that would have been impossible to justify in the 1960s. Today, trainees in psychiatry are taught to, and examined on their ability to, demarcate one illness from another, and to relate the actions of drugs to specific diagnoses. When I was trained (in Britain) in the 1960s, the teaching was that the total 'formulation' of a patient's problems and symptoms was the main aim of a psychiatric assessment; diagnosis was seen then as just a part of this formulation and not even a major part in most instances. Today, trainees in psychiatry have to be conversant with biological hypotheses (none of which has been shown to have any meaning); and discussions about treatment in clinical meetings tend to be around the sites in the brain that the drug treatment may or may not 'block'. In the 1960s biological hypotheses were on a par with social and psychological theories of 'mental illness' and generally viewed with scepticism. Today, schizophrenia, and to some extent depression, is nearly always seen as a sort of enzyme-deficient disorder; and drugs are the main, and often the only, line of treatment considered.

A point that should be noted is that the seemingly problematic nature of 'schizophrenia' as a concept is sometimes recognised and many psychiatrists are increasingly using 'psychosis' as a substitute (Boyle 2002: 247). What were regarded as 'functional psychoses' (manic depression and schizophrenia) are now seen as 'really organic psychoses that are only to be called "functional" until their organic origins are determined' (Healy 1990a: 192). Delusions and hallucinations are seen as disorders of 'form' rather than 'content', i.e. hardware problems rather than those of software (see pp. 95–6). So, psychiatrists are taught not to take an interest in the content of their patients' beliefs once the beliefs are identified as 'disordered'. In the case of auditory hallucinations, what the 'voices' tell their patients have become irrelevant, except for the purpose of 'risk assessment' (i.e. evaluating the risk posed by the content of the hallucinations). Psychiatrists seldom try to understand their patients, they merely try to diagnose them by eliciting symptoms with a series of questions, which too often tend to be standardised on the basis of data from large groups of people. Although this may seem a more 'medical' role for a psychiatrist than (what may be thought of as) a 'counselling' role, that is not really true. The approach in general medicine is increasingly towards taking an interest in the content (degrees, types, etc.) of 'symptoms' such as pain and palpitations, while psychiatrists are moving away from this approach, apparently trying to be 'scientific' doctors. So today psychiatrists and their patients carry out what historian Roy Porter (2002) calls 'the dialogue of the deaf' (2002: 156), at least as far as anyone diagnosed as 'schizophrenic' is concerned. Meanwhile, ironically, doctors in *non*-psychiatric medicine are beginning to emphasise empathy and communication.

As suggested above, the pharmaceutical industry plays an important role in promoting the trends that mark modern psychiatry as a mechanical process increasingly devoid of human feeling between persons. In the UK the Department of Health seems to promote this approach by pursuing policies of setting diagnosis-based guidelines for the treatment of 'illnesses'; at the time of writing this book British psychiatrists await such guidelines from the National Institute for Clinical Excellence. In the US, the arrival of 'for profit' managed care has led to the 'Wal-Marting of American Psychiatry' (Donald 2001: 427), decision making on therapies being based on large-scale supermarket type observations. And on top of all this the British government is about to embark on a new Mental Health Act that emphasises control and compulsion (Department of Health 2002).

I should add here that all the generalisations I have made about current trends in the practice of psychiatry do not apply everywhere and to all psychiatrists. There are undoubtedly individual practitioners who follow what are now considered old fashioned and 'unscientific' approaches in their practice. These people are sometimes referred to as 'mavericks' in the profession. The way of working that I have described as being the current scene is being promoted by various pressures that impinge on psychiatry, and by the failure on the whole for the profession to take a stand on behalf of its integrity or its patients. But then psychiatry as a body never has.

Mental health practice

An important practical feature of the mental health services today is the team approach. This allows for a variety of approaches, based on different ways of conceptualising mental distress or mental health problems, to be available to people who use the services. Yet it must be admitted that in many places it is the approach of psychiatry that dominates in two ways. First, although various models of understanding mental distress and mental disorder are presented in the training of professionals other than psychiatrists (and even sometimes in that of psychiatrists), the medical (biological) concept of 'mental illness' (which conceptualises mental health problems as being caused by pathological lesions) is the base line, or standard, that is used. Second, when it comes to actual practice in the field, the psychiatric approach overrides other approaches because of the power exercised formally and informally by doctors in the current mental health system. Of course this is particularly so at the 'hard end' of psychiatry, namely when compulsory powers are used to impose treatment, and in the forensic mental health services.

If we ignore the domination of psychiatry as described above, mental health services are no longer merely psychiatric services as they were thirty, or even twenty years ago. Various models are used within the multidisciplinary team for the understanding of what are now described as mental health problems. Dickenson and Fulford (2000), in their book on psychiatric ethics, argue that the two extremes in the variety of models are the medical (biological) and moral models; the former construes mental health problems as disorders which are matters of fact (i.e. they actually exist), while the latter construes them as matters of value. These authors believe that good practice today consists of striking a balance between these two extremes. In my view, in a multicultural setting that very balance needs to be worked out in the context of (a) diverse moralities and understandings of what mental health and mental health problems consist of; and (b) the pressures exerted by racism on the judgments made within each model and the nature of the balance.

Summary of comments on mental health services

The variety of possible approaches to mental health now available in training professionals who are working in mental health services has not resulted in a flexibility or better quality of care at ground level. The 'team' comprising, for example, an occupational therapist, social worker, psychiatric nurses and sometimes 'lay' counsellors, is invariably dominated by the medically trained psychiatrist. Although each discipline may well have had training approaches with very different emphases, the team as a whole nearly always works on the assumptions of a medical model where diagnosis is paramount. Any changes for the better (e.g. encouragement of user involvement, advent of advocacy and change from the 1979 Mental Health Act to the 1983 Mental Health Act) in the structure of the mental health services have been countermanded by changes for the worse, for example in the increase in psychiatric stigma by 'illness' being associated with dangerousness, limitations placed on professionals by rules and regulations and the advent of a 'blame culture', and most of all by the failure of psychiatry and psychology as disciplines to keep up with changes in society. In fact, my experience from working in the mental health field in England for over forty years is that the delivery of services in general, from the point of view of the user of the service, has not improved in terms of the quality of what actually matters to people who need the services. The language is different (see pp. 107–8), the treatment settings available are different (i.e. they are more community based and less institution based), the structures within which the system operates are different (e.g. clear-cut treatment plans, more formal case-conferences, etc.), but it is hard to find any improvement in terms of humanity, support and understanding, care and protection of the vulnerable, and respect for the views and wishes of service users. In addition, there is hardly any change in the appreciation of racism and cultural diversity.

What has happened in the practice of psychiatry over the past twenty years is that, under the political influence of psychotropic drugs (with the implication of specific 'cures' for specific illnesses) and the proliferation of biochemical theories about causation of the psychoses, it has swung massively into a biological mode of thought reminiscent of the German school of psychiatry of the early twentieth century. And this has happened in spite of the failure on the whole for any real 'cures' of the 'illnesses' that have been delineated, especially the 'psychoses'. Nor has there emerged any conclusions about biological or neurological 'causes' of these illnesses (least of all 'schizophrenia'). It seems that psychiatry is clinging on to Kraepelin because it has failed to come to terms with modern society, including its multicultural nature; it has failed to take on board advances in scientific thinking, including those in the neurosciences; and having lost its way in a sociopolitical morass, it seeks to maintain credibility as a 'scientific' endeavour. Yet, psychiatry remains firmly entrenched in western society and is being equally firmly imposed on other cultures.

Meanwhile, a growing scepticism about psychiatry, including its adherence to the illness model, has developed in some professionals, especially those allied to psychiatry such as psychologists, social workers and occupational therapists. However, the hold of psychiatry on mental health services is extremely strong and unlikely to diminish unless specific action is taken to change the balance of power between the professions involved in providing mental health services. Many users of psychiatric services are highly critical of the current practice of psychiatry, especially the use of medication in large doses for extensive periods, and the reluctance of professionals to refer anyone with a diagnosis of schizophrenia, for example, for 'talking therapies'. Many of these criticisms of psychiatry are general but are much more intensive in the case of black and Asian people.

Spirituality and mental health

The mental health discourse today in Europe and North America usually refers to mental health problems rather than mental illness and symptoms, but yet much of the thinking continues to be strongly influenced by ideas in western psychiatry and western psychology. These ideas are concerned with concepts built up over the years about 'mental' matters; mental illnesses, mental processes, mental therapies and so on. All the so-called information put out by psychiatry and psychology has been, and continues to be, devised within a reductionist framework, supplemented largely by a mechanistic approach of Newtonian physics (rather than modern physics). This means the reducing of complex systems into its parts, assuming that the function of the whole can be understood by analysing the functions of its constituent parts. The spiritual dimension of human beings cannot be accommodated within this approach and so psychiatry and psychology have no place for spirituality.

In their book *Zen Buddhism and Psychoanalysis*, Erich Fromm and colleagues (1960) propose that psychoanalysis emerged as an attempt, in European thinking, to find a solution to 'western man's spiritual crisis' (1960: 80), a crisis attributed by them to Europe's 'abandonment of theistic ideas in the nineteenth century' with 'a big plunge into objectivity' (1960: 79). Cultures in Asia and Africa did not undergo this change, at least not at that time; and, although undoubtedly influenced later by western ideas, appear to have maintained a spiritual dimension to their thinking in many ways until the present. Thus, it can be assumed that non-western ways of thinking accept spirituality as central to human experience, different to 'belief' or 'cognition' or even an emotional state.

The term 'spirituality', like the term 'mental health', does not denote a precise concept but is used widely. In exploring spirituality it is important to note that its essence is not necessarily represented in the written or spoken word nor evident in organised religion. In fact perhaps the opposite may be true for organised religion is more about politics and power (than about spirituality) and sometimes tends to distort, negate or even destroy the spirituality of individuals. Yet, it is true to say that wisdom within the great religions, whether oral or written, may guide one to an understanding of spirituality and spirituality may well form the original basis, the 'spiritual basis', of all religious systems and traditions. In the mental health field many people conceptualise the 'spirit' as a concept similar to the 'mind' but yet different. When people talk of being 'spiritual' they generally mean a feeling of connectedness, the personal being connected to others, the 'I and I' principle of the Rastafarians which 'expresses the oneness between two persons' (Cashmore 1979: 135), connectedness to the 'community' (a community spirit) or even wider to the land or environment (an ecological spirit?), the earth and the sky, the cosmos (a unity with 'atman' the Hindu godhead?). Lack of spirituality may be experienced as an impoverishment of the spirit, a sense of emptiness. Prayer and meditation may then be a way of replenishing this lack of spirituality; joint action in a group setting may equally well do the same and various other culturally determined ways may exist.

The first aim of this section is to provide some impressions of the cultural traditions understood as 'spiritual' that have some bearing on thinking about mental health. Ross (1992) writes about indigenous (First Nations) Americans undergoing spiritual observance in preparing to embark on a task such as making a journey or venturing on a hunting expedition. Nobles (1986) believes that the integration of mind, body and spirit is characteristic of the world views derived from African thinking and Richards (1985) makes a case for this spirituality having survived the transatlantic slave trade to continue in an African-American spirituality. Indeed Du Bois

(1970), in his classic *The Souls of Black Folk* originally published in 1904, saw 'spiritual striving' as a characteristic of the cultural ideal of black (African) Americans. Ninety years later, bell hooks (1994) writing in *Outlaw Culture*, regrets the 'spiritual loss' of modern African-American communities in the US and advocates the need for political movements that can effectively address the 'needs of the spirit' (1994: 247). It is my experience that a major demand from users of mental health services in the UK is that the disciplines of psychiatry and psychology should incorporate a spiritual dimension. This section may help to clarify what this means and how it may be brought about.

It could be stated that all religious traditions have their roots in a search for the meaning to life; the search to know, to understand, to become insightful and finally to achieve a goal. And basically spirituality means the realisation of the interconnectedness of all beings, of life as a unitary 'thing'. Then, what is seen as the 'spirit world' is part and parcel of the real world and something that is within every human being. It is likely that 'being spiritual' is implied in the process of attaining a state of salvation, nirvana or a similar equivalent ideal state that a religious system may envisage. Religious leaders and religious systems have built superstructures over the years, pointing to somewhat different paths to be followed, the languages used have differed, and their cultural contexts have been different. And of course politics (of organised religion) has distorted and often corrupted the fundamentals of every religion. However, it is possible to extract from these traditions some aspects of spirituality in, as it were, its raw form separated out from the social and political superstructures around it. Of all the great religions, Buddhism is the one that developed fairly precise methods of reaching spiritual insight and liberation from suffering. As it spread from its original source in north India to other parts of southeast Asia, China, Japan and Tibet, Buddhism accumulated varieties of practices and beliefs. However, its basic premise remains a fundamental adherence to liberation with meditation as a primary means of attaining its goals. I present here a picture of how I envisage Buddhist spirituality.

Buddhist spirituality

The term *bhavana*, or 'cultivation', is the closest Sanskrit equivalent to spirituality in Buddhist writings. Meditation is fundamental to

Buddhism and generally the means by which spirituality is experienced. *Bhavana* aims at liberating the mind and realising the ultimate truth, nirvana (Yoshinori 1995): 'The freedom attained in Buddhist practice is knowledge or reality, or rather it is reality itself, existence freed from illusions and passions that bind us to a world of ignorance and suffering' (1995: xiii). The earliest interpretations of the message of Buddhism is described by Pande (1995) as follows.

> Spiritual life consists in the effort to move away from ignorance to wisdom. This effort has two principal dimensions: the cultivation of serenity and the cultivation of insight. Ignorance is the mistaken belief in the selfhood of body and mind, which leads to involvement in egoism, passions, actions, and repeated birth and death.
>
> (1995: 10)

The wisdom through which nirvana was reached was characterised by no-self (*anatta*), impermanence (*anicca*) and suffering (*dukkha*). The variations of these characterisations, their elaborations and interpretations, resulted in a variety of Buddhist traditions. Therefore, Buddhist spirituality may seem close to what in western psychology would be seen as self-knowledge through meditation but with one important proviso. A fundamental teaching in Buddhism is the lack of a 'self' as something permanent, the 'non-selfhood of body and mind' (1995: 10), and the realisation of 'self' as illusion is an integral part of liberation. The western psychological approach of analysing the self or understanding the self, is like trying to catch up with one's shadow. In contrast to the Buddhist tradition of downplaying the self as impermanent and illusionary, western psychology elevates the self, the ego, to centre stage as something separate from all other aspects of a personal individuality, as autonomous and very important. As a result, psychological therapies, the western equivalent to 'ways of liberation' according to Watts (1971: 4), emphasise developing and maintaining self-esteem, integrity and ego-boundaries to protect the self, boost the self, etc. Similarly psychiatry (dealing with the 'abnormal') looks for abnormalities of self categorised as self-depreciation, hopelessness, guilt, etc. (Box 3.3).

Clearly there is no absolute distinction between eastern and western traditions or religious systems with respect to spirituality.

Box 3.3 Self/ego in western psychology
        and psychiatry

Separate
Autonomous
Important

Represented in psychology as
    self-esteem
    integrity
    ego-boundaries

Represented in psychiatry as
    self-depreciation
    hopelessness
    guilt
    disintegration
    passivity feelings
    dependency
    'enmeshed families'

Communication and interchange between them has not just taken place in recent times nor is it represented by the sort of 'new age' interest in eastern religions: 'Karma Cola' (to go with Coca Cola) as Gita Mehta (1980) puts it. In the introduction to a translation of the *Bhagavad Gita* (Prabhavananda and Isherwood 1947) the epic conversation between Arjuna and Krishna, which epitomises the Vedanta philosophy that underpins Hinduism, Aldous Huxley (1947), a western philosopher and scientist, states 'In regard to man's final end, all the higher religions are in complete agreement. . . . Contemplation of truth is the end, action the means.' Huxley goes on to suggest that this was a universal orthodoxy until:

The invention of the steam engine produced a revolution, not merely in industrial techniques, but also and much more significantly in philosophy. Because machines could be made progressively more and more efficient, western man came to believe that men and societies would automatically register a corresponding moral and spiritual improvement. Attention and allegiance came to be paid, not to Eternity, but to the Utopian future. External circumstances came to be regarded as more important than states of mind about external circumstances, and the end of human life was held to be action, with contemplation as a means to that end. These false and, historically, aberrant and heretical doctrines are now systematically taught in our schools and repeated, day in and day out, by those anonymous writers of advertising copy who, more than any other teachers, provide European and American adults with their current philosophy of life. And so effective have been the propaganda that even professing Christians accept the heresy unquestioningly and are quite unconscious of its complete incompatibility with their own or anybody else's religion.

(1947: 11–12)

Huxley does not mention the role of colonialism, and the racism that accompanied it and has continued even after its demise, in driving a wedge between east and west, by suppressing and denigrating eastern thinking and eastern religions and preventing, for example, eastern systems of medicine from developing. What has happened is that traditions identified in the field of mental health as western are now very different to those identified as eastern. On the whole I believe that the latter is more in line with what is generally considered a spiritual approach to life. That is the justification for my approach in this chapter to explore issues of spirituality and mental health by contrasting east and west. Yet this contrast could equally well be designated as between north and south, broad and narrow or holistic and reductionist.

In Table 3.1, I have shown the main overall differences of emphasis beween eastern and western thinking. In eastern cultures human life is conceptualised as an indivisible 'whole' that includes not just the western 'mind' and 'body' as one but also the spiritual dimension of human life, the feeling of oneness with other beings, other things even. The ideal of self-sufficiency and personal autonomy reflects a western emphasis on developing 'individuality', feeling oneself as an individual separate from others. The down side to this is that the more the sense of being an individual is enhanced the greater is the sense of 'the other', promoting the we–they dichotomy. When race is a factor for marking difference, racism is the result. In Table 3.2 I have attempted to clarify the east–west differences of emphasis a little further. Eastern traditions seem to favour knowing and understanding while the western emphasis is on gathering knowledge and analysing. Thus, for example, when some westerners go to India to seek knowledge they sometimes end up

Table 3.1 Ideals of mental health

Eastern	Western
Harmony	Self-sufficiency
Social integration	Personal autonomy
Balanced functioning	Efficiency
Protection and caring	Self-esteem

Table 3.2 Underlying eastern and western themes

Eastern	Western
Understanding	Analysing
Knowing	Gathering knowledge
Being	Having

gathering bits of knowledge rather than immersing themselves in an understanding. This difference of emphasis has been usefully conceptualised by Erich Fromm (1976) as the difference between 'having' (possessing) and 'being' (experiencing). Some psychotherapists tend to talk about having thoughts or having feelings, instead of thinking and feeling. The approach then is to objectify what is subjective in order to analyse and reduce the thoughts or feelings to their basics. This is the reductionist analytic approach that may be contrasted with the contemplative or meditative approach to understanding, understanding by awareness versus understanding by analysis (see the next section 'Treatment').

Treatment

Workers in the mental health field often see themselves as being involved in providing treatment or care for people with mental health problems – essentially thought of as problems of a personal nature traditionally conceptualised as being 'mental' or 'psychological' rather than 'physical' or 'somatic'. The concept of there being anything 'spiritual' does not come into it at all. Also, in the western tradition of psychology and psychiatry, therapy is seen as an objectified process disconnected from both the therapist who 'applies' it and the client who 'receives' it. The therapist learns the treatment and applies it within the overall medical model of dealing with problems as individual illnesses, disorders or disturbances of, what is assumed to be, 'normal' mental functioning. In an eastern

Table 3.3 Eastern and western liberation/therapy

Eastern	Western
Acceptance	Control
Harmony	Personal autonomy
Understanding by awareness	Understanding by analysis
Contemplation	Problem solving
Body–mind–spirit unity	Body–mind separation

cultural setting where such problems are seen as, say, spiritual experiences or ethical dilemmas that may or may not be medical, the process of dealing with them, or coping with the distress caused by them, is not therapy in a western sense. The usual term used may be akin to liberation (from distress) and what may be identified as techniques are more interactive alliances between people and perhaps forces in nature, rather than interventions that are objectified and separable from the person or persons involved. Looking more deeply into the process of therapy in mental health work, the western approaches are usually focused on control, of symptoms for example, or understanding by analysis, in psychotherapy for example; in other words, delineation and resolution of individual problems, whether by analysing them away or by suppressing them in some way. In cultures which emphasise harmony, balance and integration within the individual (and between the individual and others), acceptance (of problems or symptoms) is more important than control, understanding by self-awareness is more important than analysis, and contemplation is the approach of choice in contrast to focusing on the specific nature of problems. Finally in the eastern approach the whole process is carried out in a setting that addresses body, mind and spirit rather than considering each separately or excluding any part. The differences in emphases are given in Table 3.3.

It should be noted at this point, and this cannot be stated too strongly, that an approach that designates matters in the mental health field or any other field as being either eastern or western might be misleading. I have merely used these designations to indicate differences of emphasis in overall traditions, eastern and westerns traditions or 'cultures'. The differences are far from absolute, there are large areas of overlap and there is a constant interchange of ideas and views. Finally, the terms eastern and western are not meant to suggest a black–white dichotomy in any sense of the term. However, I do believe that these differences in emphasis are important because they have a significant bearing on clinical practice in western psychology and psychiatry used in a multicultural setting, with the eastern approach tending to allow spirituality to come into the picture.

As I have pointed out above and shown in Box 3.3, western psychology emphasises the self, the ego, which, unlike any similar concept in non-western cultures, is separate, autonomous and very important. Such an emphasis opposes a concept of the inter-connectedness of life, the continuity between the individual and everything else. Thus spirituality is excluded; the autonomous self is a central feature, if not *the* central feature, of all western psycho-logical theories and indeed all the therapies in psychiatry and western psychology, mainline or complementary. This self is highly personal and idealised as independent, sovereign and free; improving this self, protecting it from harm, believing in the self, defining its separation from any continuity, from spirituality, all these become the foci of therapy or self-improvement techniques. What often happens when techniques from eastern religions, or indeed gurus from the east, are adopted is that they become a means of accumulating even more knowledge or information within the self, bolstering it up, improving it, making it even more autonomous and powerful.

An emphasis on the western self, the ego, is represented in western psychology by the importance given to self-esteem, integrity and the identification of ego-boundaries. And, in line with the psychology that informs it, western psychiatry being concerned with psychopathology looks for loss of self-esteem, feelings of self-depreciation, guilt that threatens to destroy the self, enmeshment of the self (in the family) and so on, identifying these things as problems. And so medications and therapies are directed at building up self-esteem, getting rid of guilt, establishing separation of the self from the 'selves' of other people. This is not all there is to psychiatry or psychotherapy or counselling but by and large this represents the emphasis in all psychiatric and psychological therapies. And the current thinking about mental health generally reflects this.

Summary of spirituality and mental health

The meaning of spirituality in everyday work in the mental health field is often unclear, and perhaps can never be clear, but needs to be explored. That is what I have tried to do here. First, spirituality should be distinguished from spiritualism which refers to a belief in, or practice of contacting 'spirits', non-physical beings with human characteristics. Activities such as the identification of spirit possession, exorcism (of spirits) and communication with spirits during séances is bound up with spiritualism. Second, spirituality should not be equated with organised religion with a specific dogma given by a hierarchy – although it must be admitted that 'being religious' and 'being spiritual' are similar and may well be identical in some instances in some places. A western scholar of eastern traditions, Edward Conze (1957), refers to Buddhism as an 'Eastern form of spirituality. . . . Its doctrine, in its basic assumptions, is identical with many other teachings all over the world, teachings which may be called "mystical"' (1957: 11). Yet Buddhism, like Hinduism, is a system for understanding the human condition that is akin to western psychology rather than western ideas of religion. In western thinking (e.g. within anthropology) spirituality is not usually distinguished from spiritualism and is often dismissed as a belief system comprising religious ideas concerned with the soul or spirits. Traditional psychology and psychiatry take a similar approach.

These then are some thoughts and impressions that I hope are sufficiently clear to provide a sense of what spirituality means. I believe that contrasting eastern and western thinking provides an impression of how spirituality can, and should, permeate our thinking about mental health, western psychology and western psychiatry. As a psychiatrist, I can see that such a development can have an enormously beneficial effect on the practice of psychiatry, which today is increasingly impersonal and insensitive to the humanity of people seen as patients, and probably very harmful for people whose thinking is eastern; and that does not mean necessarily that they have been born in or brought up in any particular geographical area or that they are brown or black or seen as being from any particular race.

Holistic thinking

An earlier section discussed spirituality. The sort of thinking that goes along with spirituality may be referred to as 'holistic thinking', a term I use here in order to explore some of the problems that I have seen in psychiatric clinical work. These are the problems that result in misunderstandings between users of services and clinical staff, and often lead to injustice in practice. I shall start with the clinical field. The high rates of diagnosis of schizophrenia (when psychiatry is used in assessing people from non-western cultures) may arise for many different reasons. Straightforward institutional racism is one. Another problem is the miscommunication and consequent misinterpretation that comes about because of what one might call 'thinking styles'. I shall call the styles 'unconnected thinking' and 'holistic thinking' for reasons that will become obvious.

A characteristic of what is considered 'normal thinking' that underpins the practice of western psychology and psychiatry is that different events are experienced as separate from each other unless proven (cognitively accepted by the person concerned and/or others) to be connected, and that events are not necessarily imbued with feelings. In other words, events are discrete episodes and separate from feelings. I call this unconnected thinking. Also, this unconnected thinking separates out feeling, believing and knowing and even more importantly, objectifies these essentially subjective states (of feeling, believing and knowing) into 'things'; instead of the states of mind being conceptualised as ways of thinking or even behaviours or activities, they become objects 'out there' as it were that one *has*. This represents the difference between having (possessing) and being (experiencing) as conceptualised by Erich Fromm (1976) and discussed earlier (Box 3.3). Instead of seeing people as people who feel, they are seen as *having* feelings; instead of people who believe, they *have* beliefs; and instead of people who know, they *have* knowledge. This objectification of subjectivity enables psychiatrists and psychologists to analyse, measure and make judgements about, i.e. measure, objectified feelings and emotions, beliefs and knowledge.

Holistic thinking is different to unconnected thinking in being characterised by 'connectedness'. First there is a connectedness in the field of subjective feeling, believing and knowing (rather than their objectified counterparts, i.e. having feelings, beliefs and knowledge). But the primary characteristic of holistic thinking is an all-pervasive connectedness, a sort of 'connectedness thinking', that links together all happenings and experiences with feelings and instils a 'feeling' of connections between all human beings, indeed between all *beings*, and possibly between all beings and inanimate objects in the environment. Also, in holistic thinking the divisions between feeling, believing and knowing are blurred, if present at all, because these different aspects (as understood in western psychology) of thinking are connected too. Related to this feeling or cognition of connectedness may be a belief in, or rather a feeling of, pre-determination, namely a feeling that happenings are not by chance but by arrangement and there is a unity of everything animate and inanimate. In such a context, feeling something is the same as (or at least not disconnected from) believing something and all of it is encapsulated within knowing. The practical consequences of holistic thinking may be explained by the following example.

> If I meet someone who comes from a place where I lived as a child, my tendency would be to assume – although I may not be cognitively aware of doing so – that there is a connection between the meeting and the fact that the person came from the place that I was connected with. The feeling/cognition may go further in that the person's background (seen as a characteristic of the person) may be felt by me as having determined the meeting or at any rate that the meeting was pre-determined and did not happen 'by chance'.

In unconnected thinking the assumptions promoted in the above example would be that different events are unconnected (occur by chance), although if there is objective evidence to the contrary a different conclusion may be reached at an intellectual level. Holistic thinking would promote a connectedness between feeling, believing and knowing – although it would not necessarily yield an intellectual conclusion – that the events are connected. Holistic thinking is different to working out connections between different aspects of a situation. In holistic thinking all aspects are seen as one, although in practice one may separate the whole into parts for convenience in communication. Holistic thinking and spirituality are clearly allied concepts.

Of course holistic thinking and unconnected thinking in the way I have described them are two extremes on a continuum and each person goes for some location on this continuum, a location that could vary from time to time and according to context, and each culture promotes some type of mixture of the two forms of thinking. In other words, everyone is capable of both holistic thinking and unconnected thinking, of being able to connect up events and experiences 'subjectively' through feelings, and being able to analyse events and experiences 'objectively' as basically discrete unconnected matters. However, when it comes to assumptions about thinking styles in the practice of western psychology and psychiatry, unconnected thinking is considered the norm rather than holistic thinking. To put it simply, naively perhaps, correct thinking (to a western-trained psychiatrist or psychologist) is to assume that events have no feelings attached, unless proved otherwise, and feeling, believing and knowing can be objectified into 'things' that can be measured.

Mistakes in assessment

I believe that the failure of western psychiatrists, psychologists and anthropologists to appreciate holistic thinking of people and their cultures has led to serious problems both in a multicultural setting and in the practice of psychiatry and psychology in non-western cultures. Inevitably these problems are complicated by racism. Taking on the idea that Africans were characterised by prelogical thinking described as 'primitive mentality', Levy-Bruhl (1923), an anthropologist, denied that Africans have the capacity to comprehend the concept of causality and generality. While criticising this as an outmoded anthropological theory, Lambo (1969), an African psychiatrist trained in western psychiatry states:

> Reality in the western world has gone the way of attempting to master things; reality for the African traditional culture is found in the region of the soul – not in the mastery of self or outer things, but in the acceptance of a life of acquiescence with beings and essences on a spiritual scale. In this fashion only is the traditional culture mystic. Not because of any prelogical function of mind but merely because the African is the possessor of a type of knowledge that teaches that reality consists in the relation not of men with things, but of men with other men, and of all men with spirits.
>
> (1969: 207)

I believe that Lambo's description comes very close to what I have postulated as holistic thinking. Although such observations as those by Levy-Bruhl are now recognised as racist and invalid, less obvious ways in which racist ideology influences psychiatric and psychological assessments can be analysed by using the contrast between, on the one hand holistic thinking that characterises much of African and Asian cultures, and, on the other, unconnected thinking on which psychiatric and psychological cultures are based.

Generally speaking, psychiatric and psychological assessments are based on identifying and measuring various aspects of a person and putting it all together. However, one sometimes hears of 'holistic assessments', being made, usually meaning that the assessment takes on board a wide range of information about different aspects of the person being assessed: medical, psychological, social, biological, spiritual, etc. I believe that this is a mistaken use of the term holistic. Such assessments may be comprehensive but are not holistic. A holistic assessment, in keeping with the correct sense of the word holistic, implies that the assessment is done in a way that does not recognise different aspects (or 'factors') as existing separately; and that all these aspects form an indivisible whole. I believe that in making a holistic assessment, the professional must leave aside their training in professional methods of how they should go about questioning and recognising specific behaviour, beliefs, etc., and aim to get to know someone fairly intimately by listening to that person's narrative. Then the professional would be able to obtain an impression of the person's subjective feeling/believing/knowing mixture. From that an impression, a judgement, could be made of what the person needs and that is the assessment. This procedure is akin to that employed by a close acquaintance or friend but, since it is carried out by a mental health professional, the assessment would be made from an angle that brings some knowledge derived from study and experience, i.e. training. In practice the making of holistic assessments may be combined with more traditional unconnected approaches to assessment. At least, psychiatric and psychological assessments have to be sufficiently flexible if serious mistakes are to be avoided in a multicultural society. How this can be achieved will be considered in Chapter 5.

Mistakes in diagnosis

Holistic thinking can be confused with or interpreted as (the western concept) paranoid thinking or even paranoid belief. The word 'paranoid' is attached to someone's believing or thinking patterns if the cause of some happening is blamed on another person without adequate, rational reasons (i.e. objective evidence to support it). But for someone with holistic thinking to attribute blame or give credit for a happening (rather than attributing it to chance) would be a natural way of thinking. So in a multicultural society it is very important to recognise holistic thinking so that paranoid thinking is not diagnosed leading to the slippery slope that ends in a diagnosis of psychosis. It is important to note when someone is connecting events because of holistic thinking; and, if this state of affairs is leading to problems (mental health problems), psychotherapy or counselling may be the appropriate approach to take in order to enable the person to use their powers of non-holistic thinking – objective analysis of the events or experiences – in order to balance or counteract the mental health problems. An example follows.

> A person living in an area in which they feel very 'different' to people in the neighbourhood – for example because they dress differently or look different – may feel a sense of general hostility because people stare at them. Suppose that person experiences disturbance from the noise of motorcycles being revved up persistently outside their window. Holistic thinking may lead them to 'feel' that the noise is directed at them – a situation that, in psychiatric terms, could easily be interpreted as someone 'having ideas of reference'. If they then see the motorcyclists and feel frightened by (say) men in leather gear who 'look' odd or frightening, the motorcyclists may be attributed with motivations that are in keeping with previous experiences in other places. In the case of black people, such previous experiences are very likely to have involved racism. If the person concerned is disempowered – or feels a lack of control over their life – or is stressed in some other way, they may build on this feeling to the extent of feeling frightened or even persecuted.

A psychiatrist interviewing the person described above may well diagnose paranoia or even paranoid delusions. In my view this would represent an unhelpful and false understanding of what is going on. An approach that understands the meanings behind the presentation is essential for real therapy to be undertaken. Denying the reality of their experiences by, for example, saying that the person is ill is unhelpful; but helping the person to bring into play their powers of reasoning to analyse the situation objectively, i.e.

with objective thinking, could indeed help. In other words, regarding such thinking as issues around attribution (of motivations to people) or even a neurotic problem is much more appropriate than seeing it as one of paranoia. A diagnosis of mental illness, likely to be designated usually as schizophrenia or psychosis, would be both inappropriate and unjust.

Additional to the risk present in the situation described above, there is a risk that ways of diagnosing mental illness in the tradition of western psychology and psychiatry, may interpret holistic thinking as something 'pathological' in other circumstances too. Paranoid thinking (where people are blamed for trying to do harm to one while there is no reason to think so), delusional affect (where the feeling that things or people are connected when 'reason' tells one that they are not), feelings of being controlled (when one feels being controlled by forces that are external) or passivity feelings (when one feels like a passive automaton controlled by outside forces) are the sorts of thinking that may be mistakenly identified as pathological.

> Suppose A tells B that (s)he (A) comes from (say) Hounslow where B had a bad experience at one time when she was harmed by a neighbour. B would feel (through holistic thinking) that there is a connection between the two (the meeting between A and B and A's residence). The connection may just be that B thinks that A appreciates what it is like to live in Hounslow and so have sympathy with B; or it may be that B thinks that A is capable of doing some harm to B because A comes from Hounslow. The latter may be seen as 'paranoid' in western psychological terms or lead on to a diagnosis of 'paranoia' but the former (where the connection is not fashioned into a definite feeling) may not be conceptualised in that way. However, the problem is that if B tells a psychologist or psychiatrist that the meeting (in the above instance) actually occurred *because* A was from Hounslow, the psychologist or psychiatrist is very likely to diagnose a paranoid feeling, if not a paranoid delusion, or some other 'pathology' such as 'passivity feelings' or 'feelings of control', all symptoms of 'schizophrenia'. The professional may then press B with questions that push B into analysing the feeling with concrete statements about 'evidence' based on 'reason' leading B into a state of mind (as seen by the professional) that fits into a model

of illness that the professional is comfortable with (in non-holistic, reductionist thinking).

Grier and Cobbs (1969) in their classic book *Black Rage* described '"healthy" cultural paranoia' as a coping mechanism used by black people in a context of widespread racism in the US: 'He must maintain a high degree of suspicion towards the motives of every white man and at the same time never allow this suspicion to impair his grasp of reality' (1969: 135). Psychologist and psychotherapist A. J. Franklin (2002) finds that black youngsters in the US need what he calls 'healthy suspiciousness' in order to survive and so sometimes need to be taught, for example, the skill of being suspicious of the police without provoking a hostile response when, for instance, they are stopped while driving a car. A. J. Franklin sees it as a function of a therapist working with black boys to ensure that they have this skill.

I know of black people in Britain who feel that they are constantly being watched, for example by means of closed circuit television (CCTV) cameras fixed at many street corners, a reflection of 'cultural paranoia', and when under stress find it difficult to maintain a grasp of reality because the fact is that CCTV cameras are indeed commonplace now in many parts of London where black people live. I believe that for black people living in a racist society, suspiciousness of people around them is an understandable state of mind. Unfortunately, this sort of suspiciousness may well be interpreted in a criminal justice context as an indication of guilt of an alleged offence, and in the psychiatric or psychological system as pathological paranoia. It is only a small shift in thinking, a shift that is very easily made by holistic thinking, for a person who has dealt with life's problems by means of 'healthy paranoia' to believe that a range of devices are being used to spy on them, and/or that a wide range of people are following them about. If they come up against a psychiatrist with little understanding of the reality of their lives, paranoia or even paranoid schizophrenia or psychosis may be diagnosed. Professionals who do this are not necessarily racist, they are merely trying to make sense of what they see and hear using the system of psychiatry that they are used to and modes of thinking inherent in the system. It is the system they operate that is racist. This is institutional racism.

In summary, I believe that the tendency for psychiatric and psychological ways of diagnosing paranoia can be traced to the failure to appreciate or take account of holistic thinking. When this occurs in a context of racism, and when professionals do not appreciate the experiences that people have in society and/or do not understand the coping skills that they have to use in order to survive, serious mistakes can be made and pathological paranoia diagnosed inappropriately. It is then only a small jump to a diagnosis of schizophrenia or psychosis. The issues outlined above are taken further in Chapter 5.

False and true beliefs

Interpreting beliefs is an important part of psychiatric expertise. In its reductionist approach psychiatry and to a large extent western psychology aim to categorise beliefs, usually into true and false beliefs. Yet, the judgement as to whether a belief or set of beliefs is true (and justified) or 'false' (and unjustified) is basically based upon interpretations of the human world, world views, appertaining to the beliefs in question. In other words, the nature of belief is mainly determined by culture. Also, the process of 'developing' beliefs, really the nature of thinking along certain lines, is tied up with ideologies held by people and communities, social construction of language and a host of other dimensions of the human condition. An important part of a psychiatric system is to designate some beliefs as 'delusions' – false beliefs of a certain type – and such designation underpins the diagnosis of psychosis. In fact, the genesis of beliefs, how and why people believe in something, is a complex matter, something that psychiatrists and psychologists are seldom qualified to understand. Yet, psychiatrists and psychologists are called on to make judgements about people's beliefs, separating normal beliefs from pathological beliefs (i.e. 'delusions'). I do not have the knowledge or space in this section to cover adequately the diversity of the literature on belief and thinking that may be relevant to psychiatry and western psychology. However, I have selected some pointers from modern neuroscience as possibly helpful in getting some understanding of how delusions should be viewed.

In his well-known book, *Descartes' Error*, neurologist Damasio (1996) has written about the integrated (holistic) functioning of the brain and body. Damasio suggests that for effective social and personal behaviour individuals have to 'form adequate "theories" of their own minds and of the minds of others' (1996: 174).

Charlton (2000) uses Damasio's ideas and others to develop a critical approach to psychiatry based on modern neuroscience and biology, an approach that can be applied clinically. Charlton proposes that the sort of beliefs that are identified as delusions, 'boil down to beliefs about agency – the power and influence of powerful and influential agents – whether human or supernatural' (2000: 28). Delusional disorder is diagnosed when such delusions are present in a chronic and 'encapsulated' form (encapsulated meaning limited to a few situations or people), while the person's speech, emotional reactions and general behaviour are not seen (from a psychiatric standpoint) as abnormal in any way. 'In other words a person with a delusional disorder is essentially normal except for the subject matter of their delusions' (2000: 28). The mechanism by which beliefs are developed are seen by Charlton as 'social intelligence', reflecting social pressures.

In discussing the diagnoses 'schizophrenia' and 'delusional disorder', Charlton (2000) distinguishes two kinds of delusions: 'bizarre delusions' and 'theory of mind' delusions. 'Social intelligence interprets behaviour in the light of inferred *mental states*. In other words, the mechanism of social intelligence makes "theories" of mind, which are inferences about what other people are thinking – their motivations, intentions and dispositions' (2000: 30, italics in original). 'Theory of mind is the name given' by Charlton following Damasio (1996) 'to the ability of humans to make inferences ("theories") about the contents of other people's minds' (Charlton 2000: 17). According to Charlton, bizarre delusions arise when there is clouding of consciousness from some organic cause such as brain disease, injury or drug effect. 'In lay terms, all individuals with bizarre delusions will be overtly 'mad' or in some other way suffering from brain impairment' (2000: 47). The beliefs which he calls 'theory of mind delusions' are a part of normal life; they come about as a result of a person making inferences by 'reasoning logically from false premises' (2000: 39), using his/her own emotional reactions as indicators. He points out that these inferences may be attributed to whole categories of people, rather than to individuals. The beliefs may be 'false' but they are not associated with clouding of consciousness or indeed any other 'symptoms' apart from what are seen (in psychiatric terms) as 'delusions'.

'Delusional disorder' is a diagnosis given to people who have beliefs judged to be 'false' but not associated with other symptoms. The beliefs are 'theory of mind delusions'; their basic falsity lies in the premise from which the beliefs derive. So a person who is seen in psychiatric terms as suffering with delusions of persecution would be someone who attributes the motivation of persecution to a person (or persons) who behaves (behave) in a certain way. The research in exploring delusional thinking as problems arising from attribution is mixed (Boyle 2002). But there is some support for the suggestion that paranoia is basically a reflection of attributional style of people (deemed 'paranoid') in making judgements about social situations (Bentall *et al.* 1991). It is suggested that people deemed to have persecutory delusions are likely to attribute the source of life events to other people than to circumstances (Lyon *et al.* 1994). Certainly, my own clinical experience is consistent with this view. When people seem to have beliefs that appear to me to be 'false' I try and help them to understand the nature of the derivation of their beliefs, how they have come to make attributions that lead to the beliefs. And of course these attributions are made in a context and the context may play an important part in the genesis of the premise and so the beliefs themselves.

In psychiatric practice today, delusional disorder is often subsumed within 'schizophrenia' and people who, strictly speaking, could be diagnosed as suffering from delusional disorder are given the label 'paranoid schizophrenia'. In my experience, this habit is particularly prevalent in the case of black people. It is very common for black patients, especially those in forensic hospitals, to be called 'paranoid schizophrenics' where the only symptom is paranoia, often related to issues around persecution by people in authority, or white people in general. Taking Charlton's approach, the basis of the diagnosis is that the premise (upon which various beliefs have been developed) is what is false. And one needs to see how this premise may have developed. Admittedly, unravelling the nature of a false premise may be complicated but it is preferable and much more sensible than merely designating the belief as a delusion and stopping there.

In a context where a person or group of people is/are generally picked upon, persecuted or oppressed for illogical reasons (such as skin colour), the falsity or truth of the premise becomes problematic. Many black people have developed strategies for countering racism, or at least not letting racism influence very much their ways of thinking about people in general. However, there are bound to be people who do not cope so well or who, when under pressure (from say being discriminated against overtly) or when depressed as a result of some misfortune or illness, think in ways that are 'false premises'. They may then attribute causation for social events to external forces. The premises that they may come to may be, for example, that the police are after them or that neighbours are making a noise to drive them out from their home. Such beliefs may become the subject matter of a belief that could dominate a person's life or at least become so important that the person talks about their beliefs in order to get something done about them. In current psychiatric jargon the beliefs themselves are seen as the symptoms, symptoms of paranoia yielding a diagnosis of paranoid schizophrenia. But given the general context of society (i.e. what goes on in society in general), the premise in terms of its meaning may be an exaggeration but cannot be deemed to be false. The designation of psychosis may well be inappropriate and damaging. This theme will be taken up in Chapter 5 to suggest a way forward within the psychiatric illness model.

Psychotherapy and counselling

The origins of what are currently referred to as psychotherapy and counselling started with Freud and developed as 'psychodynamic therapy' in the nineteenth and early twentieth centuries in mid-Europe. Littlewood (1989) puts it succinctly: 'Freud's innovation was to unite in a single idiom both phylogenetic [evolutionary] and individual development, generating an evolutionary model which traced our development as persons in parallel with the conjectural psycho-history of humankind in general' (1989: 10). And this was in the nineteenth and early part of the twentieth centuries when (in European thinking) there was no recognition of any valid history apart from European history and where racist images of so-called black, brown, yellow and red people, images informed by ideas from social Darwinism of higher and lower races, were accepted as scientific truth. It was a context where people thought of as racially non-European were held to be inferior and savage, primitive and underdeveloped. It was inevitable in such a situation that when psychologists and psychiatrists encountered people perceived as not white, analogies were drawn between the primitive non-European and the neurotic (e.g. Freud), between dangerous-ness of black people and repressed unconscious feelings of white people (e.g. Jung), and so on. And so myths and stereotypes of black, brown and yellow people were incorporated into psychological and psychiatric theories and practices.

Early in the twentieth century, Freud (1913) saw similarities between 'the mental lives of savages and [European] neurotics' in his book, *Totem and Taboo* (1913: title page); Jung identified a 'very characteristic defect in the Indian character', i.e. 'deception' (Jung 1939: 524); and Devereux (1939), an anthropologist, viewed non-western healers (generally referred to as 'shamans') as neurotics or psychotics. The first textbook that addressed issues about psychopathology in non-Europeans was written by an eminent president of the American Psychological Association, Stanley Hall (1904); in it he had a whole chapter about 'adolescent races', referring to Asians, Chinese, Africans and indigenous Americans. The image of black (and other non-white) people as culturally and biologically 'underdeveloped' people has persisted ever since, underpinning psychiatric and psychological thinking, and assumptions that affect psychotherapy and counselling practice. In the 1930s Jung, hypothesising that evolutionary development led to 'historical layers' in the brain (analogous to the anatomical layers of the brain cortex), concluded that the '"Negro" has probably a whole historical layer less' (Thomas and Sillen 1972: 14). In analysing Jung's writings, Dalal (1988) concludes that Jung equated the white person's unconscious with the black person's conscious, and then assumed that what he could discern of his own unconscious life represented the symbolism used by black people 'It is certain that Jung feared the black man. . . . His error was in assuming that because the blacks symbolised the primitive to himself, therefore they were primitive' (1988: 13). In a similar way, the stereotypes that influence modern-day therapists often link up with their own fears and anxieties, and end up re-enforcing them.

Although psychotherapy began with Freud and his psychodynamic school of psychology, there are many schools of psychology today that inform various types of psychotherapy and counselling. But psychologies from non-European cultural traditions are ignored almost totally and the developmental model from psychodynamic theory is usually basic to most training in psychotherapy and counselling. However, since psychotherapists and counsellors work with people from a diversity of cultural backgrounds, questions about cultural relevance must apply to many of the ideas and assumptions that therapists work with. Even more importantly 'subtle racism' through institutionalised attitudes and assumptions influences the therapeutic relationships that are an essential part of psychotherapy and counselling.

Transcultural issues

There are many issues around ways of thinking implicit in psychotherapy and counselling that need to be considered in a transcultural perspective. Issues centring on the concept of 'self' implicit in western psychology are discussed earlier in this chapter. Most therapists give importance to 'self' in understanding the 'inner world' of a client, see the aims of therapy as the development by the client of insight into aspects of their 'self', understanding blocks to the development of such insight, etc. Yet, 'self' is neither fixed nor rigid as many psychotherapy systems, especially those dependent on development theories, assume. As Littlewood (1989) says: 'We use different aspects of our personhood in different situations' (1989: 9). In a multi-ethnic society the context in which a person lives is culturally complex and affected by racism. Therefore the therapist dealing with a black client must be conversant with the client's world, either through experience or as a result of training that enables him or her to obtain this understanding if therapy is to be sensitive to the client's needs. Furthermore the aims of therapy assumed by the therapist or counsellor are often very different to those assumed by the client, differences determined at least partly by cultural background (Fernando 1995c). For example, many western approaches emphasise the attainment of personal autonomy as desirable while in other cultures the emphasis may be on harmony and interdependence; similarly a problem-solving approach may be less important in non-western cultural traditions where the approach to problems may be to contemplate their complexity (see pp. 121–2).

Another problem in applying psychotherapy and counselling transculturally arises from the implications of what therapy itself is all about. This is also referred to earlier in this chapter. Western approaches in general are usually focused on managing an internal life eliminating, for example, symptoms, neurosis or psychosis through understanding by analysis. In Asian cultures the emphasis is on the development of harmony and balance through liberation from, what may be seen as, despair or suffering; and understanding by contemplation supersedes understanding by analysis (see Fernando 1995c). The east–west differences depicted in Box 3.3

and Tables 3.1–3.3 (pp. 121–2) indicate how difficult it may be for a therapist or counsellor to transcend cultural gulfs between therapist and client. But that is what therapists and counsellors have to do if they are working in a multicultural society.

When we come to actual practice, an issue that is often ignored in psychotherapy and counselling is the politics of the encounter between therapist and client or, more broadly, between the institution that the therapist works in (community centre, social services office, voluntary project, etc.) or adheres to (analytic psychotherapy, intercultural therapy, etc.) on the one hand, and the client on the other. A client may see the institution as white or even racist, or as medical rather than psychological, etc. So what clients tell therapists in a particular setting may be very different to what they tell some one else in a different setting, and to some extent this is irrespective of the nature or orientation of the individual therapist or counsellor. In one situation somatic idioms may be used and in another psychological or sociopolitical language. The whole approach to self-disclosure is a complex matter anyway and depends, among other matters, on how the client perceives the therapist. Issues around power, expectations and fears play their part. Racism and cultural difference influence all these matters.

Ethnic-specific services

In the UK, especially in London, there are many organisations in the black voluntary sector (Chapter 1) that aim to provide psychotherapy or counselling for people from black and Asian communities, and indeed other minority ethnic groups. The therapists in many of these ethnic-specific services (some of which are described in Chapter 1) claim to provide therapy that is 'not eurocentric' (personal anecdotal information). However, what this means is far from clear, especially as many of these therapists state that their training was largely 'eurocentric' in nature. Unfortunately, this topic has not been investigated in any depth although there have been several publications, listed in Chapter 5, describing ways in which psychotherapy and counselling should change in order to suit the needs of a multicultural society.

Some parts of the US too have seen the advent of ethnic-specific services providing psychotherapy and counselling but, there too, studies have not gone beyond outcome studies, which incidentally support the usefulness of ethnic-specific services (e.g. Lau and Zane

2000). But a preliminary and limited study of how these services may differ from traditional western services is reported by Ito and Maramba (2002). When Asian-American therapists (Asian-American meaning Americans of East Asian, mainly Chinese, origin) working at an ethnic-specific center in Rosemead, California were asked in a systematic qualitative study 'what they thought they were doing and what they thought their Asian-American clients and the clients' families assumed' (2002: 64–5), a very complex picture emerged. In contrast to that at traditional western services, therapy at this center seemed to be characterised by negotiations and modifications between therapists and clients, accommodation of families in the therapeutic process, an approach to issues of dependency that did not tally with traditional views on 'counter-transference', and the promotion of personal relationships between therapists and clients. Many therapists at the ethnic-specific center felt comfortable in their interactions with clients in a way that they had not felt when working in a traditional western mental health service; and they reported that in the traditional western service (but not in the ethnic-specific service) they often felt intimidated and pressurised to behave in ways that jarred with their natural inclinations. Some of this rings true for the UK too. Many therapists working in ethnic-specific services in the UK tell me that a major factor that aids the therapeutic process is that both they and their clients feel safe in the ambience of an ethnic-specific service, while, in generic settings, there is a certain tension around them and their clients. In my view, this tension reflects the racist pressures that abound in society as a whole and permeates many ordinary mental health settings. I believe that this fact alone is a powerful argument for providing ethnic-specific mental health services.

Asian traditions

Concepts of illness and treatment, as well as those of health, that pervade most of south Asia are based on traditional Ayurveda as described in the writings of Susruta and Caraka, collected in the *Susruta Samhita* and the *Caraka Samhita*, partially translated into English (Susruta 1963; Agnivesa 1983). Traditional Chinese medicine is undergoing a revival in the west as an alternative to western medicine but in China it is increasingly being used in conjunction with western medicine. Hence, in this chapter I explore the approach to therapy in the eastern tradition by considering Ayurveda and traditional Chinese medicine in south Asia and China respectively.

Ayurveda

The most popular system of indigenous medicine in India and Sri Lanka is Ayurveda, which literally means the science of life. Mental hospitals in India and Sri Lanka, modelled on western mental hospitals, were introduced during the colonial period and still function. Also psychiatry and western psychology have been promoted as disciplines and so people trained as psychiatrists and western psychologists practise in both the statutory and private sectors of health care. However, indigenous systems of care exist side by side with these western methods of therapy for mental health problems. In my own experience, it is relatively common for people in Sri Lanka and India with mental health problems to consult both Ayurvedic physicians and western-trained psychiatrists. Indeed in most countries of south Asia it is commonly the custom for people to use multiple therapy systems (see Nichter 1980; Sachs 1989) and in the case of what in the west are called 'mental health problems' this would include indigenous non-medical healing (see Amarasingham 1980; Waxler 1984). On the whole, therapy for mental health problems would sometimes be covered within the Ayurvedic system, while indigenous religious systems of therapy may well be resorted to when someone is considered 'mentally ill'. Traditionally, Ayurveda recognises forms of madness given the generic term *unmada*. The use of religious healing ceremonies, including exorcism rituals, predates Ayurveda in the Indian tradition; these and other ways of dealing with *unmada* due to spirit possession 'stand out as an uneasy meeting between medical and priestly concerns' (Kakar 1984: 248).

In considering Ayurveda, we have to note that ideas within the system are mingled with those of Indian philosophy and psychology, ritual and religion, in what Obeyesekere (1977: 155) calls 'a metamedical extension of medical concepts'. Further, Ayurveda is as much about 'dissertations on correct behaviour' as about medical treatment and prophylaxis, and, from the psychological angle, Ayurveda is a 'repository' of Indian cultural thinking about the human body and the concept of the person (Kakar 1984: 220): Diagnosis in Ayurveda is very complex; it is really an assessment that includes causes (*nidana*), premonitory indications (*purvarupa*), symptoms (*rupa*) and full extent of the disease (*samprapti*) (Jaggi 1981). To know the stage of the disease is important from the therapeutic point of view, because the same medicine is not useful or may even prove harmful when administered at the wrong stage of the disease. Also, the deduction of the patient's personality type is part of an Ayurvedic diagnosis. All this is perceived in relation to the qualities that are traditionally expected, and (as in western psychiatry) social desirability is equated, more or less, with health. In an Ayurvedic assessment the patient's constitution includes his/her mental state (or state of mind), judged against a norm that rests within Indian philosophy and religion. 'Normal mind (*satva*) consists in memory, veneration, wisdom, valour, purity, and devotion to useful work' (1981: 144).

The essence of healing in Ayurveda is integration and balance; all disease involves psychological or emotional imbalance and Ayurveda has methods for enhancing mental as well as physical well being.

> For healing of the mind, it employs various yogic and spiritual therapies including meditation, mantra, prayer, visualizations, and rituals called 'spiritual therapy' (*daiva cikitsa*). [But] Ayurveda also employs its regular physical healing means and modalities to treat mental conditions. Moreover, a pattern of imbalance on the mental level, with disturbed thoughts and emotions, is usually reflected and reinforced on a physical level.
>
> (Frawley 1989: 247)

The treatment in Ayurveda for 'mental' disorders is not differentiated from that for bodily illness; and there is no systematic theory of 'mind' and 'mental' processes as there is in western thought, although some forms of therapy for 'restraining the mind' derive from the various schools of yoga. In addition, 'purification' by purges and enemas and 'pacification' by decoctions that tranquillise, counteract depression and strengthen the nerves may be used (Kakar 1984). While western psychotherapy is rooted in the western tradition of introspection aimed at knowing oneself and characterised by scrutinising 'events' and 'adventures' of one's own life (Simon and Weiner 1966), the Indian tradition of examining one's self is characterised by meditative procedures of self-realisation. The 'self' of Indian thinking is 'uncontaminated by time and space' (Kakar 1984: 7) while the western 'self', explored by introspection, is made up of deeds and emotions set in history.

In practice, Ayurvedic physicians in, for example, Sri Lanka do not treat everyone who is suffering from 'mental illness' (in western terms). Most people deemed 'psychotic' in western terms might well be treated by exorcism or some other form of what may be called 'religious therapy'. Indeed, Ayurvedic physicians may work in conjunction with such therapists. Exorcism rituals in the Indian tradition predate Ayurveda, and these religious ways of dealing with madness due to spirit possession 'stand out as an uneasy meeting between medical and priestly concerns' (Kakar 1984: 248), as they do in the west. The difference is that, in practical terms, they are not in conflict, one merges into the other. And neither Ayurveda nor, for example, Tantric healing, an equivalent of western psychotherapy, is secular in the way that western psychiatry and psychology are secular. Neither recognises an absolute distinction between mind and body nor sees an individual as distinct from the total environment, the cosmos.

Classical Ayurvedic treatment (when seen from a western point of view) is basically physical; but then the mental and physical are not considered as two separate things or structures, as they are in western medicine. In one part of the *Caraka Samhita* (Agnivesa 1983: 231), a classic Ayurvedic text, therapies are divided into three general types: 'Spiritual therapy, therapy based on reasoning (physical propriety) and psychic therapy'. The first and last are clearly 'psychological' in the western idiom. Spiritual therapy includes incantation of mantras, wearing of talismans and gems, making auspicious offerings, as well as what may be called religious activity such as the 'observance of scriptural rules, atonement, fasts, chanting of auspicious hymns, obeisance to gods, going on pilgrimage, etc.'; and psychic therapy is described as the 'withdrawal of mind from harmful objects' (1983: 231). All three types of therapy are recommended for most diseases.

Chinese medicine

A variety of medical systems, conforming to a basic pattern and based on an understanding of the human condition that reflects Chinese philosophy and tradition, especially the Taoist concept of yin and yang, is generally called Chinese medicine. The *Nei Ching*, the classic text of medicine in this tradition, has been translated into English as *The Yellow Emperor's Classic of Internal Medicine* (Veith 1966) since it has been attributed to the Yellow Emperor. According to Hammer (1990), in the early 1960s the Chinese government brought together a group of acceptable Chinese physicians and ordered them to create 'traditional Chinese medicine' as a uniform system of medicine. Today, traditional Chinese medicine is practised in general hospitals throughout China side by side with western medicine. Often patients seek both concurrently and are encouraged to do so. But China, like other non-western countries, has mental hospitals modelled on the lines of western mental hospitals. In modern times, people identified as 'mental' tend to be admitted to these hospitals that are run very much on the lines of western mental hospitals. In these hospitals, traditional Chinese medicine is not applied at all and the approach they seek to emulate comes from western psychiatry. Psychology (western psychology) as such is still virtually unkown (at least that was the case when I visited China in November 2001) and so the concept of psychotherapy is still strange to most Chinese health professionals in China. However, in the time of Mao Tse Tung, a hospital in Shanghai was said to have used 'heart-to-heart talks' as a part of therapy (Ratnavale 1973: 1084). At present, western psychotropic drugs seem to be the only therapy available to people classified as 'mentally ill' in China. However, many people with (what may be identified in western terms as) mental health problems may well be seen in general hospitals and clinics and treated with a mixture of traditional Chinese medicine and western medicine. Unlike in India and Sri Lanka, indigenous religious modes of therapy for mental health problems seem to have been suppressed together with the suppression of all forms of religious activity since the advent of communist rule in China. At least, even if these systems of therapy are still used by Chinese people, very little is known about the extent to which this takes place.

Kaptchuk (1983), a western authority on Chinese medicine, states 'The logic of Chinese Medicine is organismic or synthetic, attempting to organise symptoms and signs into understandable configurations. The total configurations, the patterns of disharmony, provide the framework for treatment. The therapy then attempts to bring the configuration into balance, to restore harmony to the individual' (1983: 4). Thus a Chinese doctor would identify 'heart disharmony', 'lung disharmony', 'spleen disharmony', etc.

A disharmony would be further analysed in terms of deficiencies or excesses related to the yin–yang balance. Thus, the excess or deficiency of various emotions are recognised and related to disharmonies located in various organs.

> It is only when an emotion is either excessive or insufficient over a long period of time, or when it arises very suddenly with great force, that it can generate imbalance or illness. And the reverse is also true: Internal disharmony can generate unbalanced emotional states.
>
> (Kaptchuk 1983: 129)

According to Hammer (1990), Chinese medicine classifies the aetiology of disease into three main categories: 'Foremost of these is the "emotions", the "Internal Demons": anger, grief, fear, joy, compassion, anxiety, and worry.' . . . Internal Demons are responsible for alterations in the energy system of a person, affecting to one extent or another the mind, the body or the spirit' (1990: 20).

In traditional Chinese medicine theory, body, brain, spirit, mind and the rest of the human condition are indivisible. As with Ayurveda, from a western viewpoint traditional Chinese medicine is somatic rather than psychic. But Hammer (1990) believes that from a western viewpoint traditional Chinese medicine can be seen as being entirely psychological, having a similar basis to psychotherapy. In practice, the therapy administered by a traditional Chinese medicine physician covers advice on ways of life and diet, together with herbal remedies, massage and acupuncture. The exact mixture would depend on the type and form of disharmony to be counteracted (Kaptchuk 1983). All the types of therapy, whether they are seen as physical or psychological 'advice' (in western terms) have both spiritual and bodily effects as seen from a western standpoint.

Summary

The medical approach to madness evident in Hippocratic medicine of ancient Greece was elaborated in the Arabic Empire (between the tenth and thirteenth centuries AD) when mental hospitals first appeared. But the origins of modern western psychology and psychiatry can be traced to the sixteenth century when knowledge about the 'mind' (psychology) and disorders of the mind (psychiatry) was built up against the background of Cartesian duality. Concepts of 'degeneration' and 'atavism' played important roles in the construction of 'schizophrenia' at the turn of the twentieth century. Although the practice of psychiatry has changed over the years, it remains tied to a (western) illness model for understanding mental health problems. And recent trends tend to promote psychiatry as a mechanical process devoid of human feeling.

In this chapter it is argued that cultural traditions that emphasise spirituality give rise to what is described here as 'holistic thinking'. The failure by western psychology and psychiatry to take account of cultural diversity in forms of thinking is a serious drawback in a multicultural setting. Furthermore, in a context of racism, this failure may give rise to mistaken identification of pathology. This is particularly so when psychiatry attempts to identify false beliefs in what it calls 'delusional disorder'.

The concept of 'self' is an important aspect of psychological theories that underpin psychotherapy and counselling. Yet, cultural differences in the way 'self' is perceived and experienced are seldom taken on board in practice. Nor is it common for counsellors and psychotherapists to address the nature of the encounter between therapist and client in the context of racism. Finally, this chapter considers briefly some Asian traditions with respect to health and illness, to illustrate the variations that exist in the connections between philosophy and religion on the one hand, and mental and physical aspects of human beings on the other.

Chapter 4

Psychiatric stigma and racism

The term stigma denotes a marker, either visible or implied, that discredits a person or group of people (Goffman, 1968). However, the marker itself carries baggage of its own in terms of feelings, attitudes and historical happenings. It is not just people, or groups of people, who are affected by stigma but stigma may be attached to a diagnosis of illness; stigma with respect to a psychiatric diagnosis is called 'psychiatric stigma'. In the past the main illness that was stigmatised was leprosy – interestingly in western but not in non-Western cultures (Fabrega 1991b) – and more recently AIDS has been stigmatised. Many psychiatric diagnoses are stigmatised but the main object of psychiatric stigma today is schizophrenia (Cannon 2001).

There is a long history of racism in western culture (Chapter 1). Sometimes racial designations have become stigmatised and used in order to disempower and oppress people. Thus, the designation 'Negro' was such a term. Often racial designations collect baggage to become terms of abuse, or at least ones that imply disparagement of some sort. 'Coloured' is such a term in Britain today, but possibly not in some other places such as Canada where 'people of color' is an acceptable description of certain groups of people. Being called black used to have a stigma in the US until this was reversed by the Black Power movement of the 1960s. Of course, racial groups are not all stigmatised but the words used in racial descriptions often have implications because of the context in which they are used. Thus, what is often implied in western countries when people are referred to as white and non-white is that the latter lack something that the former have, that non-white people are deficient in some way – the context being one of white supremacy. In a similar vein, the state of being white is assumed to be a pure state that is contaminated by genetic mixing with black people – represented in the nineteenth-century American definition of black people as people who had at least 'one drop' of 'black blood'. This stigmatisation of racial difference can occur in other contexts too. The word 'Turk' has at least two meanings in the English language according to *The Oxford English Reference Dictionary* (Pearsall and Trumble 1995); 'a native or national of Turkey' or 'a ferocious, wild or unmanageable person' (1995: 1551). We may not think directly and consciously in terms of dictionary meanings of words, but this double meaning indicates how assumptions are woven into our common sense, how our perceptions of people can be biased, and how, in this case, referring to someone as a 'turk' implies stigma. However, it must be admitted that the stigmatisation of a racial designation is variable, depending on the way racism is manifested in the society concerned.

Writing from the point of view of people who suffer psychiatric stigma (people given a stigmatising diagnosis of mental illness), Crass (2000) examines what actually happens in practice. She argues that the focus should shift away from 'stigma' attached to mental illness or people diagnosed as suffering such illness, replacing its discussion with language of prejudice and discrimination. In a similar vein, Sayce (2000) believes that the notion of stigma individualises what is really societal discrimination. Indeed, psychiatric stigma is essentially discrimination against people who are given a psychiatric diagnosis. Racism, too, involves discrimination, in this case usually on the basis of skin colour. Both discriminations may be expressed overtly in terms of personal prejudice or subtly through institutional processes (see Chapter 1). Although I see the value of abandoning the notion of psychiatric stigma for the reasons given above, I prefer to stay with the notion of stigma in the light of the primary purpose of this chapter, which is the exploration of the reasons why racism in mental health services and psychiatry seem to persist as a powerful force in spite of the prolonged struggle against it (Chapter 1).

Introduction

The concept of stigma has been written about extensively within psychology and sociology (see Jones *et al.* 1984; Crocker *et al.* 1998). A recent analysis from a psychiatric viewpoint is one by

Haghighat (2001). When a psychiatric diagnosis is stigmatised the victims are the people who happen to have been given the diagnosis, usually by psychiatrists but also by others. The popular use of the term can tell us quite a lot about the way stigma works. For example, it is not only people that are referred to as 'schizophrenic' but attitudes of mind, national policies, etc. are referred to as 'schizophrenic', always in order to denigrate. The very word 'denigrate' means 'to blacken' according to *The Oxford Reference Dictionary* (Pearsall and Trumble 1995: 381), an example of how racist images have been incorporated into the language.

People designated as schizophrenic are, at the least, discredited by and, at the worst, socially excluded by society as they are considered to be alien, or foreign, to what is considered normal society. So, psychiatrists in nineteenth-century Europe, being responsible for designating who was mentally ill (and hence alien to society) and who was not, were called 'alienists'. When a racial group is stigmatised people perceived as belonging to that group also face problems of social exclusion, and in extreme instances they are seen as alien to society in the same way. So, early twentieth century legal moves to limit immigration to Britain was an 'Aliens Act', and when The Netherlands decided in 1994 to impose sanctions on airline companies carrying some immigrants to the country the law brought in was also an 'Aliens Act'.

Both psychiatric stigma and racism are based on certain hypotheses or assumptions. In the case of mental illness, it is assumed that that there is an objective 'thing' called 'mental illness' that affects the person given the diagnosis; in the case of 'race', that the concept 'race' has validity for differentiating one person (or group of people) from another person (or group) on a variety of dimensions. Therefore, countering stigma in either instance necessarily means countering the corresponding assumptions. Both psychiatric stigma – especially that attached to either the diagnosis of schizophrenia or the more general 'psychosis' – and racism are closely involved with the exercise of power. To designate someone as a 'schizophrenic' or a 'psychotic' invalidates everything they do or say, it designates them as 'alien' to society, not to be trusted, not to be taken seriously. Racial designations used as stigma ('he's coloured', i.e. not quite right) carry similar baggage for similar reasons. These designations carry images of alienness, fear, dangerousness, deceit, etc., that come to us from a historical background, stereotypes, our own (sometimes subconscious) fears and prejudices, and so on. However, the people stigmatised may sometimes evoke positive feelings too; in the case of schizophrenia ones of sympathy and understanding and, in the case of race, attraction or even fascination. But the predominant images and feelings in this day and age evoked by both schizophrenia and racism are mainly negative ones. The point is that racism and the diagnosis of schizophrenia both carry immense power in western society for a myriad of reasons. Exploring these can shed light on how the stigma in both instances persists, and such an exploration could help in understanding how we can deal with the problems of racism in psychiatry.

In 2000, the Royal College of Psychiatrists embarked on (what it called) an 'anti-stigma campaign' calling it 'Changing Minds: Every Family in the Land' (Crisp 2000). The campaign is ostensibly aimed at counteracting psychiatric stigma by focusing on publicising what it saw as the medical reality of mental illness as being treatable by psychiatrists. Underlying this approach is the view that stigma is a barrier to providing care for people who need treatment for mental illness and a source of social exclusion and discrimination against the mentally ill. However, some users of psychiatric services object to the campaign because, by its very nature of emphasising bio-logical pathology as causing psychological problems and medical treatment as curing them, the campaign promotes stigma. The argument here is that stigma is an inevitable result of promoting modern biological psychiatry, a view supported by some psy-chiatrists (e.g. Chaplin 2000; Summerfield 2001).

Fabrega (1991a) has reviewed and analysed the recent history of psychiatric stigma in western societies. He concludes that discredit is attached to psychiatric diagnoses in the same way that it is attached to incapacity and institutionalisation (because they enable people to opt out of being productive), but that psychiatric diagnoses are linked also to disapproval in society because the illness may not have an objective marker, suggesting feigned disability. Thus, psychiatric stigma in the modern era derives from both 'isolation and alienation promoted by chronic institutiona-lization' (1991a: 116) of the mad or insane (i.e. today's 'schizo-phrenic' or 'psychotic') as well as the blame attached to someone who may be feigning illness. So, while I concede that psychiatric stigma is not a simple issue, the fact that stigma is inherent in the meaning of schizophrenia to both psychiatrists and the general public – in other words, in the common sense of western culture –

renders it difficult to argue that one could aim at removing stigma while keeping schizophrenia just as it is.

Prevalence of psychiatric stigma

Fabrega (1991b) writes that psychiatric stigma seems to occur in many societies, both eastern and western, but points out the difficulties in analysing exactly how, and to what extent, psychiatric stigma occurs in very different cultural settings. For example, since most non-western cultural traditions handle illness in an integrated way without differentiating it along psychiatric versus non-psychiatric lines (as in the west), the matter of stigma attached to psychiatric illness is difficult to evaluate. Further, there is variation in the way psychiatrically ill (as seen through western eyes) people are handled: 'Some are medicalized and stigmatised, some are not, creating a picture that is complex because of true cultural variability and the fact that the Western bias about "the psychiatric" is not found' (1991b: 548). Warner (1983) has questioned whether stigma as identified in the west is all that prevalent in the 'Third World'. And Littlewood (1988) has argued, rightly I think, that 'generalising about cross-cultural differences in psychiatric stigma is premature given the paucity of knowledge' (1988: 1057).

I can add a personal note here. When I visited Sri Lanka in 2000, I had the opportunity of speaking with psychiatrists practising there and also with some of the social workers who had been visiting relatives (living in the villages) of patients institutionalised for many years in a mental hospital near Colombo. The psychiatrists generally believed that these patients had been abandoned in hospital by their relatives because of stigma. However, the social workers, speaking in Sinhala, told me that relatives did not generally see these patients as being outcast or alien as implied in the word stigma, but as people needing care and help – and very often they (the relatives) were unable to provide this care. What I heard ties into my own recollection of how 'mad' people were seen in Sri Lanka. Generally, especially in communities that had not been westernised, madness was viewed as an affliction that affected someone, a 'possession' in western terms. Once the person's affliction was relieved, they may need care but the negative labelling of madness disappeared. The observations in Sri Lanka by anthropologist Nancy Waxler (1974, 1979) support my view. Waxler (1974) writes about what she calls traditional societies:

The sick person, himself, is not believed to be responsible for the illness; his body or soul may be possessed but his 'self' remains unchanged. If he follows the appropriate prescriptions, then it is believed that his symptoms will disappear and he will quickly and easily return to normal. There is no stigma attached to mental illness; no one believes that the patient is 'different' and should be treated in a new way after his symptoms have gone.

(1974: 380)

In a later publication, Waxler (1977) writes: 'mental illness in traditional societies is often thought of simply as a misfortune, a discomfort, a problem that deserves care and treatment, but not as shameful or something to hide' (1977: 243).

In Sri Lanka, as in many traditional (i.e. non-western) societies, indigenous medical healing, western medical healing (including psychiatric therapies) and ritual or religious healing (mostly, in the case of mental health problems, applied to people that western psychiatrists would designate as being 'psychotic' or 'schizophrenic'), all exist together. People pick and choose one or the other, or more often access two, or all three, systems at the same time. In writing about the progression of a patient suffering from mental illness in Sri Lanka, anthropologist Amarasingham (1980) states that Ayurveda (an indigenous medical system), ritual treatment (e.g. exorcism) and western medicine (psychiatry) have 'interlocking historical roots . . . [leading to the development of] . . . underlying coherences' (1980: 88). In effect, in Sri Lanka very different world views about the aetiology of mental illness or madness have become integrated into a complex whole. Shame and stigma about 'madness' do exist but, in my view, they exist to the extent to which mental illness is perceived as familial, a view that comes mainly from western influence. In view of the difficulties in considering stigma internationally and across cultures (see pp. 150–1), the discussion on psychiatric stigma in this chapter will be limited to the situation in western societies, namely those in western Europe and North America.

Stigma, discrimination and schizophrenia

Stigma is perceived as an attribute of people who are stigmatised, 'an attribute that is deeply discrediting' (Goffman 1968: 13).

However, it is not a fixed attribute but one that is variable, sometimes reversible, and always arbitrary in that the reasons for the attribute being present are never clear. Although stigma is generally conceptualised as an attribute of a person, a group of people or a 'thing' such as an illness, Goffman (1968) has made the point that 'a language of relationships, not attributes, is really needed' in understanding stigma (1968: 13). In other words, stigma is a reflection of the way people relate to one another or the way society relates to a person or group of people. Essentially, 'the process of stigmatisation revolves around exclusion of particular individuals [or groups of people] from certain types of social interactions' (Kurzban and Leary 2001: 201). And exclusion implies discrimination through individual (or group) prejudice or institutionally mediated processes. Frable (1993) has proposed two dimensions of stigma, namely danger and visibility, as mediators of the reactions (of society in general or other people) to those who are stigmatised. Others (e.g. Jones *et al.* 1984) have suggested several other dimensions, but Frable's two dimensions would do for our purposes. Frable's suggestion means that the extent or power of the stigma relates to the perceived danger (of the person or 'thing' having the stigma) or the degree of visibility of the stigmatising mark. In the case of psychiatric stigma the person stigmatised as a result of the label 'schizophrenia' or 'psychosis' is certainly perceived as dangerous in some way but may not be all that visible. But in the case of racism, skin-colour racism in particular, visibility is unavoidable. In fact, it is often the case that the greater the visibility, the greater the power of racism.

Discrimination is closely related to power. The ways in which power is exercised in any society is complicated but identifying one or more groups that need control is always a feature of the exercise of power. The history of psychiatry shows that the need to diagnose mental illness was intimately tied up with the need to control populations and people (Chapter 2), i.e. the exercise of power. Over the years, the power of psychiatry has become integrated with the power of the 'state', the power of the system that is in control and wants to remain in control. This is exemplified very clearly in the case of so-called 'political abuse' of psychiatry in the former Soviet Union (Bloch and Reddaway 1984), which is discussed later (pp. 160–1). A similar situation occurred in apartheid South Africa. Apart from the (white) South African State practising apartheid in patient care and staff appointments, resulting in inequality of mental health care based on race, Smith Mitchell and Co., a white-owned company run for profit, provided custodial 'care' under contract to the government for 10,000 to 20,000 black patients. A delegation from the American Psychiatric Association (Stone *et al.* 1979) visited South Africa in 1978 and reported on the 'enormous discrepancy between white and black facilities . . . [and that] the decision to transfer patients to Smith Mitchell facilities [was] predicated on the economic constraints dictated by apartheid' (1979: 1505). What was called 'industrial therapy' in the Smith Mitchell Institutes included the maintenance of buildings and subcontracting of patient labour to other firms (Leading Article 1977). The shocking thing was that the all-white Society of Psychiatrists of South Africa made no attempt to counteract the racism of its psychiatric services. It even claimed that 'very extensive and advanced psychiatric services [are] given to all South Africans without reference to colour or creed' (Gillis 1977: 920–1).

Just as diagnosis is a reflection of the exercise of power, so is racism. And within the psychiatric system, race power and psychiatric power have intertwined. Racism has, as it were, permeated psychiatric stigma rendering diagnostic thinking to become racist thinking. The ways of diagnosis promote racism. For example, when schizophrenia is 'found' to be commonly diagnosed among black people in a particular setting (e.g. inner cities of Britain) being a black person in that particular setting becomes a signifier for the diagnosis. If an illness is commonly found in a particular group then one gives priority to it in that group. In the BBC's *Horizon* programme called 'Black Schizophrenia' (referred to in Chapter 2), Dr Lambo, the eminent Nigerian psychiatrist, pointed out the danger of studies such as the one on which that programme was based, namely the one by Harrison and colleagues (1988). (This study was one of the early studies to find a very high rate of schizophrenia being diagnosed among African-Caribbean people: the findings of a high incidence of schizophrenia were presented without any critique of the meaning of diagnosis and the subjective nature of identifying symptoms on which diagnoses are based.) By generalising about racial groups examined in a narrow context (in this case by using a diagnostic tool that does not have proper validity) racist assumptions can be re-enforced; in this instance the assumption was about black people being violent and genetically inferior (the stigma carried by the image of schizophrenia). Thus the power of psychiatry operates through the common sense of ordinary people and ordinary psychiatrists. In the context of mental health today, schizophrenia is a major player in the exercise of power, so it is necessary at this point to examine the case of schizophrenia as a diagnosis.

'Schizophrenia' as a diagnosis

The effect of psychiatric stigma is to enable society to discriminate against people given a psychiatric diagnosis such as schizophrenia because then such discrimination seems to be given validity. After all, it could be argued and is often assumed that this is a medical condition which we know (*sic*) is associated with dangerousness, violence, confusion and, more than anything else, alienness that renders people who are afflicted with it as being beyond under-standing, irrational, bizarre, etc. But why is this? What is so powerful about the marker schizophrenia? One way of examining this is to consider the historical origins of schizophrenia (see Chapter 3, 'Medicalisation of madness and distress').

From the very beginning of its construction, schizophrenia, together with eugenics, was a product of race thinking, represented in Morel's theory of degeneration (amplified by Lombroso in 'atavism'). This ideology was absorbed into the Nazi movement that tried to get rid of degenerate races, degenerate art, and so on. Together with this link to racism, schizophrenia was constructed to encompass criminality and inherent inferiority. It is not surprising therefore that schizophrenia carries a stigma, nor that the label of schizophrenia carries racist implications. In a way, that is what is it is supposed to do, to imply degeneracy, racial inferiority and criminality. And when present-day psychiatrists draw on the Kraepelinian tradition and diagnose schizophrenia that is what they do too, although admittedly many do not realise it. More than that, the negative labelling carried by schizophrenia has spread to the more general diagnosis of psychosis because in modern times (in Britain at any rate) the two labels are used almost synonym-ously. The case against schizophrenia as a diagnosis is now very strong and is considered briefly in the rest of this section.

The historical context in which Kraepelin constructed schizo-phrenia (as 'dementia praecox') as an 'illness' was discussed in Chapter 3. Although generally accepted as such, the diagnosis 'has remained a persistent source of controversy and uncertainty' (van Praag 1976: 481). In a paper in the *Lancet*, Hays (1984) is highly critical of Kraepelin's original approach in identifying a unitary psychosis in the asylum patients (identified by Kraepelin as psychotic) who were not suffering from manic depression. Sarbin and Mancuso (1980) point out that 30 years of research has failed to produce a marker that would establish the validity of schizophrenia as an illness. And, writing from a background of many years of researching schizophrenia, Johnstone (1999) refers to 'the central difficulty of the lack of an effective validating criterion [for schizophrenia]' and 'the lack of clarity of any underlying process' (1999: ix). Psychologist Richard Marshall (1995) rejects any scientific basis for the concept schizophrenia as representing illness.

> The 'illness' notion on which schizophrenia is based is at the level of metaphor or analogy. It is simply a result of an analogy with organic illness. It is metaphorical thinking – it is *as if* what is termed schizophrenia *is* illness, a result of organic defect. . . . From a true scientific viewpoint, then, an illegitimate and unwarranted assumption has been made. We have moved from the realms of science and into the reaches of belief.
>
> (1995: 57, italics in original)

After analysing the concept schizophrenia in terms of its construction, its diagnostic criteria and its genetic research, psychologist Mary Boyle (2002) comes to the conclusion that abandoning it would enable the study of 'phenomena' (that at present are linked together into an illness which is assumed to have a 'cause') in their own right, taking on board 'questions about context, about content and function and about social and personal meanings' (2002: 245). Another psychologist, Richard Bentall (1990), after reviewing the evidence on reliability and validity of schizophrenia as a clinical diagnosis in western settings, concludes that the 'current faith in the scientific meaningfulness of the schizophrenia diagnosis cannot be justified' (1990: 32). The concept of schizophrenia as an illness has not shown itself to be useful for purposes of biological research. One reviewer of the topic (Barnes 1987) concludes: 'For every point about the biology of schizophrenia there is a counterpoint. Theories about the origin and disease process of schizophrenia are often built on a multitude of empirical observations and a paucity of hard facts' (1987: 433). Another review (Lieberman and Koreen 1993) finds a 'fragmentary body of data which provides neither consistent nor conclusive evidence for any specific etiologic theory' (1993: 371). In yet another, Jenner and colleagues (1993) conclude:

> In our opinion, what all these studies [of schizophrenia] appear to indicate is that the finding of (more or less conspicuous) neurobiochemical, psychophysiological, psychoendocrinological, or neurophysiological anomalies (when we proceed to study the working of the human brain) does not necessarily imply the existence of any sort of disease process (which could therefore be the only one capable of producing the anomalies).
> (1993: 106)

McGorry (1991), a psychiatrist, and Charlton (2000), a psychologist, both arguing from a neuroscientific perspective, believe that using the concept 'schizophrenia' is actually impeding psychiatric research and preventing therapy for people with mental health problems. And Bentall and colleagues (1988) attribute the lack of any substantial progress in schizophrenia research in a century to schizophrenia not being a meaningful scientific concept.

It was noted in Chapter 1 that the use of schizophrenia as a diagnosis for international research by the World Health Organisation (in its *International Pilot Study of Schizophrenia* – IPSS) has been strongly criticised by Kleinman (1977) – a criticism echoed by others (e.g. Marsella 1982; Favazza 1985; Fernando 1991). And I argue in this book and elsewhere (Fernando 1988 1998b) that the use of schizophrenia as a diagnosis is no longer useful in a multi-ethnic society. But worse than that, black people, and black communities as a whole, experoence the diagnosis of schizophrenia as oppressive. Some comment on the way diagnosis is made in psychiatric practice may be appropriate at this point.

Making a diagnosis

In psychiatric practice (unlike in general medical practice), symptom identification and illness recognition are not independent processes, the former following the latter; in psychiatry they occur *concurrently*. As Kendell (1975) pointed out many years ago, decisions about diagnosis are made early in a clinical interview, before the psychiatrist makes judgements about the presence or absence of symptoms. Thus, images that the psychiatrist has in his or her mind about the sort of person who is likely to be schizophrenic, for example the alienation that the psychiatrist feels from the thought processes of the supposedly 'schizophrenic' patient, and what schizophrenia is associated with, for example a sense of fear in other people, affect the psychiatrist's judgements about the presence or absence of symptoms and signs. During recent years the diagnostic process for identifying schizophrenia has become standardised, with structured ways of eliciting and recording symptoms and operationally defined criteria for diagnosing the illness; the most popular criteria for diagnosing schizophrenia being 'first rank symptoms' (Schneider 1959). However, the basis on which this superstructure has been built remains weak since it is largely a matter of the judgement by one individual about emotions, behaviour and feelings of another. When a psychiatrist identifies 'phenomena' such as delusions or thought disorder, he or she is actually interpreting feelings and beliefs – these phenomena are not something 'out there'. As Berrios and Chen (1993) note, calling them 'phenomena' implies that these judgements are objective facts. In other words, as Fulford and colleagues (1993) point out, evaluation of human features in the process of making diagnoses are inevitably value laden, and on the whole the values come from the culture within which psychiatry has developed and the culture in which it lives and breathes, both reflecting western values and western perceptions about culture, race, etc. The issues around identifying psychiatric 'phenomena' are discussed more fully in Chapter 1.

Since diagnosis in psychiatry is largely a matter of making judgements about people, it is unavoidably open to bias and prejudice. The use of operational criteria for identifying schizophrenia as an illness (now a standard procedure in research) may help to overcome idiosyncratic diagnostic habits and increase reliability of diagnosis but, as researchers Wessely and colleagues (1991) admit, in reporting a study of the Camberwell Case Register, the use of such operational criteria 'brings us closer to committing Kleinman's "category error"' (1991: 798). In any case, standardised methods are seldom used in clinical settings and so even this limited safeguard against inconsistency does not operate in clinical work. So, whether standardised methods are used or not, the context in which diagnosis takes place is all important. I have argued in earlier chapters (especially in Chapters 1 and 2) that the British context is imbued with racism. Racist myths and stereotypes dominate thinking whether one likes it or not; and the background to psychiatry and psychology, and its failure to counteract racism in its institutions, means that institutional racism is rife.

However, racism enters the diagnostic process at other levels too. After all, diagnosis is always based on a personal interaction involving at least two people. In such an interaction, images of black people must play a large part in the conclusions drawn about diagnosis, and such conclusions inevitably affect interpretations that get classified as symptoms. Particular diagnoses carry particular images and the images about illness get confounded with images about people. For example, alienness is an attribute we see in people we consider to be aliens or foreigners and much of this feeling is connected with how people look, i.e. their 'race'. But alienness is also linked to images of the mad, the people beyond the fringe, the schizophrenic. Further, when there is a view of schizophrenia as being caused by a 'bad' gene (a view that is deeply imprinted in psychiatric thinking) the idea of genetic inferiority gets linked to schizophrenia, while the ideology that sees black people as genetically tarnished is not an uncommon concept that informs thinking about race anyway. This confounding of alienness and biological or genetic inferiority with race, and with schizophrenia would promote a diagnosis of schizophrenia among black people. In my view, it is not necessarily a '*mis*-diagnosis'; it is the application of an inappropriate and unhelpful, even destructive, label used within the tradition of psychiatry.

When I was training in the 1960s, I was taught that 'West Indians' presented with primitive psychoses rather than clear-cut illnesses in the European mould. Even then I noted the slippage of meaning of the term 'primitive' applied to both illness and to people. Many of the stereotypes that inform our attitudes in diagnosing are connected with the sort of racist ideology that associates skin colour with primitiveness and often with dangerousness and even madness. A black woman once told me in describing her efforts at self-control 'I am not allowed to be eccentric, if I do something outrageous it is seen as madness – as schizophrenic.' Just as some American psychiatrists saw runaway slaves as suffering from drapetomania (see Chapter 1), it is not difficult to understand how angry or frightened 'aliens' (i.e. black people) may be seen as suffering from schizophrenia or psychosis (this is discussed more fully in Fernando 1998c).

Finally, an aspect of diagnosis in current clinical practice is its relationship to treatment. The traditional view is that treatment is determined by diagnosis, and therefore correct (*sic*) diagnosis is essential. In my view this is seldom the case. The cynic, looking at the way most psychiatric systems work, may conclude that a psychiatrist generally decides on what treatment should be given and then makes a diagnosis that fits in. In my view that too is seldom the case. Although diagnosis plays a part in determining treatment, decision making is far more complicated in practice. If we consider the case of someone who is agitated and perhaps frightened, and even angry, the context in which the psychiatrist makes the treatment decision is fraught. Here, the difference between treatment and control is likely to be very unclear. So if one wishes – or thinks it prudent – to give high doses of psychotropic medication because the patient seems to need 'control', the schizophrenia diagnosis, or at least a psychosis diagnosis, becomes imperative. Black people get caught in these situations much more often than white people do; but even more importantly, stereotypes and images play havoc in such situations and again being black plays into the schizophrenia diagnosis.

Summary of schizophrenia as a diagnosis

I put forward here a case against the use of schizophrenia as a diagnosis. First, there are problems with the concept of schizophrenia when considered from a historical perspective – its emergence as a 'new' construct in the early 1900s, its dubious validity even in terms of methodology at that time, and its construction in a context of racist eugenic thinking dominated by the ideology inherent in the concept 'degeneration'. Second, the concept of schizophrenia has not proved useful as a basis for research into understanding mental health problems from a biological viewpoint; its use in international study (i.e. in the IPSS) has been unsuccessful in that results of studies have confused rather than clarified issues around therapy for, and outcome of, mental health problems. Third, when looked at transculturally, schizophrenia does not stand up as a useful way of identifying mental ill health; some of the symptoms considered to be cardinal signs of illness, such as 'hearing voices', may not be thought of as pathological in some cultures. Fourth, schizophrenia does not seem to mean very much as an explanation for mental health problems to either service users or to their carers and relatives. Fifth, the use of medication, often in high doses, is not necessarily related to a diagnosis being made first, therefore the separation of the diagnosis from the therapy would clarify the reasons for using medication in patients who are agitated and thereby reduce its abuse. Finally, when 'schizophrenia' as a diagnostic concept is used in a multi-ethnic setting, many problems emerge; in Britain it has become conflated with racist oppression, raising questions about the racist nature of the diagnosis itself in conjunction with psychiatric stigma. One cannot but conclude that the usefulness of schizophrenia as a concept denoting illness is now unsustainable and its relevance in a multi-ethnic society is suspect.

Racism and power

Racism in society is reflected in the mental health field by racism in psychiatry (see Chapter 1). It is worth considering how this has come about in Britain. Since the 1950s Britain has experienced the loss of its empire. This has resulted in the decline of direct power over colonies inhabited by black people but an influx of these same black people, and indeed others who identify as black, into Britain. The empire has, as it were, come home to Britain. Sociologist Stuart Hall and others pointed out in the 1970s that this migration of black people was recognised by British society as a threat, and the control of black people became a political aim, although never voiced explicitly (Hall *et al.* 1978). This control is no longer at arms length (in far flung colonies) but right here in Britain itself in, as it were, internal colonies (Hall *et al.* 1978).

In the 1960s a strong movement grew up protesting at the so-called 'abuse of psychiatry' in the old Soviet Union (Bloch and Reddaway 1984). In short, some political dissidents were being sent to secure hospitals, especially the Serbsky Institute in Moscow, having been diagnosed as schizophrenic because of their bizarre behaviour, delusional and grandiose ideas, etc. One thinks of a similar situation in the time of slavery in the US when some runaway black slaves were diagnosed as suffering from drapeto-mania (mania for running away). Foucault (1988) has pointed out that during Stalinist times, psychiatry in the Soviet Union had a very low profile. It was with the liberalisation of the political system under Khrushchev that so-called abuse of psychiatry occurred. Actually it was not really 'abuse' as much as the 'use' of psychiatry for control and domination. It is likely that many of the diagnoses made were perfectly respectable within the psychiatric medical model. The people who were sent to hospital were, in terms of Soviet society, irrational and unrealistic, they did have ideas that psychiatrists within the Soviet system could well have interpreted as delusional.

In Britain today excessive numbers of black people are being diagnosed as schizophrenic and being sent to secure hospitals and units (Chapter 1). In a context of racism where the control of black populations is clearly on the political agenda (although not stated overtly), the analogy with what happened in the Soviet Union in the 1960s is obvious. Psychiatrisation has become a tool of racism, or rather racism has been implemented through psychiatry. Of course it is not straightforward and psychiatry works through processes such as stereotyping, on the basis of images and myths that I have already discussed in Chapter 1. For example, the 'big, black and dangerous' image was identified in the inquiry into the deaths of black people in Broadmoor Secure Hospital (Special Hospitals Service Authority 1993) as an important factor in determining diagnosis and seclusion (solitary confinement) in British forensic psychiatry. Also, more general issues such as the association of both blackness and schizophrenia with violence, the medicalisation of social problems allied to power, the pharmaceutical firms peddling medication as a cure for all such illness, etc., are all involved in the power that is exercised over black people through the psychiatric system. But clearly, psychiatry is in effect being used for internal colonialism. This is not say that all psychiatrists are personally racist or colonialist. Just as some Soviet psychiatrists in the 1960s may have been secret service agents, some psychiatrists may well be prejudiced. However, it is the working of the psychiatric system that I am alluding to as being racist. The trouble is that because of its very nature, its lack of much objectivity, its dependence on common sense and poor validity of the criteria used in diagnosis, psychiatry has always been – and as far as I can see always will be – open to permeation by social and political forces and so easily used to promote whatever power is dominant in society.

Blaming the victim and biological thinking

In Chapter 3, I describe the recent changes in psychiatry in western Europe and North America, noting a marked swing towards a biological mode of thinking. The result is not just a shift in practice with emphasis on biological causation and biological therapies (i.e. drugs) but a shift in training of psychiatrists as well as that in the disciplines allied to psychiatry, such as social work and psychology. In this context, one has to appreciate the power of psychiatry in underpinning the thinking about mental health, influencing the agenda for mental health policy and determining the way people perceived as suffering from mental illness are dealt with. The increasing power of stigma is understandable: it is part and parcel of reversal to nineteenth-century Kraepelinian thinking. Why has this occurred? The answers are too complex to be analysed fully here but one general factor within western society may be highlighted.

In Chapter 2 it was seen how the race riots in Bradford and Oldham were attributed to the failure of the Asian population to integrate and live in the same areas as white people. 'White flight' (i.e. white people moving away as Asian people move into a previously white area) and racial harassment of Asians are discounted. This is victim blaming. In Britain today, the blame culture has caught on to such an extent that if anything untoward happens to someone who is a psychiatric patient it is assumed that 'someone' else *and* the 'patient' concerned have to take the blame. All over western society there has been a shift towards (as a British prime minister once said about a new approach to criminality) more blame and less understanding. Blaming the victim, when transposed to the mental health field, becomes the application of a stigmatising diagnosis. We see this very clearly in the way schizophrenia is used today. It is not 'just' an illness but also a designation of foreboding, fear and dread. Something to be controlled. In many instances it implies some sort of racial danger and hence the need for control of black people or black communities. This is partly a hangover from the Kraepelinian era (see Chapter 2) when it was constructed as something that reflected the dreaded inherent degeneration with its racial connotations, the very 'thing' that was later controlled by murder and genocide of degenerate races. In the political field of social and health policy, blaming the victim leads to identifying faults in people, rather than social or political systems, to explain disorder, criminality, etc., and to develop policies 'on the hoof' based on soundbites rather than organised thinking.

The manifestation of racism in Britain's multi-ethnic society has changed since the 1980s (see Chapter 1). The changes have affected the language used, it has become less overtly abusive but disempowering. The changes have also resulted in a differential application whereby street racism persists, and may well have increased, while overt racism directed at professional classes has decreased; in a strengthening of institutional racism in the face of attempts by the government to minimise overt prejudice through legal means; and finally in accentuated racist thinking associated with the so-called 'war against terrorism' launched by the US and Britain after the attack on New York in September 2001. All this has reverberated in the mental health field in ways that I have described in Chapter 2. Thus, racism works through stigma, power and discrimination within psychiatry and mental health services. I believe it has much to do with the shift that has occurred in psychiatry itself – especially the shift into biological thinking – and with the baggage that psychiatry carries in its diagnostic system.

The power of racism in society at large hitches on to psychiatric diagnosis of schizophrenia with ease. The struggle against racism in mental health services is fraught. Racism appears to hide within psychiatric stigma – so much so that service users may mistake racism for psychiatric stigma and vice versa – and they become almost indistinguishable from one another in practice. Indeed, my experience of attending discussions in which white service users participate, is that many white service users tend to deny the importance of racism, attributing all the problems suffered by black and Asian people within the mental health services to the disadvantages derived from being seeing as mentally ill, i.e. to psychiatric stigma. In the British professional arena, the amalgam of fear instilled by the stereotypes associated with black people and Asian people, of psychiatric stigma, of assumptions of white supremacy and of the impulse (even responsibility) to control degeneracy provide a basis for racist practice. I shall illustrate this with my experience of a case conference at a major teaching hospital in east London.

One day in late October 1996 I had just finished giving a lecture to trainee psychiatrists at a London teaching hospital when a black trainee (possibly the only one in the group who really appreciated what I was driving at in my talk on racism in psychiatry) invited me to attend a case conference in the Department of Psychological Medicine. There were about 30 people present – psychiatrists, social workers, psychologists, and trainee psychiatrists. A white female student presented the 'case' and a black male psychiatrist chaired the meeting. The student read out the history of the patient whose 'case' was being presented. He was described as a black man who had been charged with actual bodily harm to a woman. The student then showed a picture of a white girl with blond flowing hair stating 'This is the girl who he was found to have harmed.' It was noted that this alleged behaviour was the sole 'symptom' that the 'patient' suffered from. The alleged offender had not touched the alleged victim but merely looked at her, having followed her to her place of work. The verdict of guilty that the court had found was unprecedented in such circumstances but the man had been turned over subsequently to the psychiatric system for 'observation'.

In the discussion that followed three senior psychiatrists argued with one another about a possible diagnosis of De Clérambault's syndrome (a condition where someone believes that another person is in love with him/her). A black trainee pointed out the social class discrepancy between the alleged offender and alleged victim but his comment was ignored. A white junior psychiatrist wondered why the 'patient' had been charged at all and commented 'perhaps it's because this man is black'. A black psychiatrist said that in an earlier case when a black man was charged with actual bodily harm towards a black woman he was found not guilty because he had not touched her. A white social worker who had never met the patient commented twice 'I really feel frightened of this man. He could murder someone next.' A white senior psychiatrist said that race was very important here and that the case reminded him of Clunis: 'It's just the murder that is lacking.' [Clunis is a black man who had stabbed a white man at a railway station believing the latter to be persecuting him. The matter was the subject of an enquiry (North East Thames Regional Health Authority and South East Thames Regional Health Authority 1994)]. The black psychiatrist chairing the meeting was uncomfortable throughout the discussion and tried to turn the discussion away from race by pointing to a directive on risk assessment issued by the Royal College of Psychiatrists, but to no avail.

The Professor of Forensic Psychiatry (a white man who is often consulted by the British Department of Health) who had been present throughout the discussion was asked for his opinion. A hush descended – this was clearly the final word, the pearls of wisdom. He said that when he heard that a psychiatrist from a Special Forensic Hospital was visiting the patient he had rushed after that visiting psychiatrist to ensure that he recommended sectioning 'If he was dealt with by the law he would have got a couple of years and we had to ensure that he was put away for ten or twelve.' ['Sectioning' in Britain refers to compulsory detention in hospital under a 'section' of the Mental Health Act.] To the professor, the question of diagnosis was secondary. When I questioned the ethics of his action comparing it to what happened in the Soviet Union in the 1960s when psychiatrists put people away compulsorily because they were considered dangerous to society, the learned professor commented 'Well what would you have done . . . we have checks and balances – there are the tribunals and so on to make sure there is no injustice.' A white female clinical psychologist–psychotherapist commented 'After all what you did was to get him somewhere where he would get treatment.' Several of her psychology colleagues nodded. The white staff clearly found it a good case conference. The black staff, including the psychiatrist chairing the meeting, were silent. I exchanged meaningful looks with the student who had invited me to attend the case conference.

The case conference I describe above is typical of case conferences in the field of forensic psychiatry. On this occasion the undertones of racism were obvious to me but what really surprised me was the lack of insight into their own reactions among the people who spoke up, especially the white female psychotherapist and her (white female) colleagues, and the clear disempowerment of the black staff, including the person who chaired the meeting. Race was certainly discussed, but as an interesting side issue. Ethics, culture, power and social exclusion were not even referred to. And the medical implications of the diagnosis, and the diagnosis itself, were secondary to the underlying agenda of control. Naturally, the diagnosis was schizophrenia. One question that stayed with me after the meeting was: how can black professionals help black patients in such a situation? But the question that is pertinent to this section of the book is: what did this man suffer from – stigma of mental illness or racism?

Summary

Stigma has always been closely associated with the concept of mental illness developed within western psychiatry, and is attached to many of the diagnoses within psychiatry, especially to psychosis and schizophrenia. Although the reasons for this may well be complex, the reality for users of mental health services is that psychiatry itself is felt as oppressive in many instances. Racist thinking has become implicit in many diagnostic formulations and thence has fed into the information that underpins mental health services. The fact is that racism has been very resistant to all efforts to reduce its power in the practice of psychiatry. The argument I make here is that its persistence is partially explained by the permeation of racism into the diagnostic process and thence its integration with psychiatric stigma. This is especially so in the case of the diagnosis of schizophrenia and the more general psychosis.

We can understand how this has come about by examining the way schizophrenia was constructed as an illness at the turn of the nineteenth into the twentieth century. Schizophrenia was the epitome of Morel's concept of degeneration – a tendency to revert back to a primitive racial type – that lies dormant in white people and may be manifested unless prevented from doing so. It follows that the dormant nature of this tendency would be unsustainable if the person is black to start with. The drive to prevent degeneration from manifesting itself led to the killing of schizophrenics and then to genocide of people held to belong to degenerate races in the first half of the twentieth century. Even before that, racial inferiority was a reason put up to justify slavery of black people by white people. It seems that society has slipped into using schizophrenia to justify oppression in the latter half of the twentieth century and the early twenty-first century.

I concede that one may argue that themes prevalent in the past need not necessarily determine what happens today. Unfortunately, society and psychiatry has changed in such a way as to promote, not retard, oppression through psychiatry. Changes in society have predicated emphases on competitiveness and self-interest; a tendency to see the human condition in biological terms; the quick fix; and the need to blame someone when there is some misfortune. All this, taking place in a context where individual responsibility (and hence blame when something goes 'wrong') is emphasised, gets reflected in the psychiatric field by a strengthening of categorisation, a reversion to Kraepelinian concepts of racial degeneracy interpreted as an inherited tendency where the diagnosis of schizophrenia or psychosis becomes a calling to account, and the perpetuation of stigma carrying racial undertones and overtones. Racism and psychiatric stigma have blended together to exercise power over black people. Psychiatrists are caught up in this; mental health services serve as the vehicle for it.

Part III

Changing practice

Chapter 5

Moving forward

The need for change in psychiatric practice and delivery of mental health services is now acknowledged widely. Confronting ethnic issues (Chapter 1) is acknowledged as a priority, if only by implication, in the National Service Framework for Mental Health (Department of Health 1999) referred to in Chapter 2. I believe that the long-term answers to the problem of addressing cultural diversity and counteracting racism in psychiatry and mental health services are in making fundamental changes in psychiatry and psychology in conjunction with changes in society at large. In the case of psychiatry, it has to move away from its adherence to the narrow biological model, 'Kraepelinian' or 'neo-Krapelinian' psychiatry' (Chapter 3), that it has slipped back into recently. Indeed, there has been a shift of the biomedical model in general medicine towards a biopsychosocial model (Engel 1977) and some doctors, including some psychiatrists, have already moved towards this. But that is not enough. As Harari (2001) points out, psychiatry must be practised in a way that appreciates 'the clinical and ethical limitations of concepts derived from simple empiricism' (2001: 729). This means that, in a multicultural world, the discipline has to be opened up to concepts of mental health from all cultures and it has to identify and counteract racism in its practices, its theories and its research.

Notwithstanding the above, I believe that it is unrealistic to expect – or even try to achieve – a sudden revolutionary change in the practice of psychiatry and thence to the training of psychiatrists. Yet change must come and so consideration must be given to strategies to achieve change. I suggest that in the short term, the struggle is to enable services to be more 'culture sensitive' and minimise the effects of institutional racism. On the face of it

this should be a fairly simple matter. But the reality is very different. The field of cultural diversity itself has many ramifications
when one tries to apply it in service provision; and counteracting
racism is far from simple. Much has been written on both these
matters and this book adds to this literature. The main fact to bear
in mind is that there are no simple answers. Therefore, it is very
important for anyone devising strategies for change to be informed
by a range of opinions and views of people both in the voluntary
and statutory sectors, including a range of service users. The
temptation to depend on the ability of one or two persons to devise
a strategy, though seemingly an easier option, may well be
counterproductive. This chapter presents a few suggestions for
moving forward. These are only *my* views, informed by limited
experience and based on the arguments presented earlier.

A cry that is often heard when the need to move forward is
raised, is for training. In fact, training in 'race and culture', 'cultural diversity' or 'transcultural psychiatry' is often designated as
the most important part of any strategy to meet the problems that
underlie ethnic issues. But to judge from the failure in most
instances to look at the outcome of training (to see whether race
and culture training results in changes in practice) my impression is
that far too often institution of a training scheme is resorted to as a
way of getting out of changing practice. This is not to say that race
and culture training provided for mental health professionals is to
be condemned. Such training is important and valuable. And there
are some good schemes, for example that incorporated in the
document prepared for the Department of Health, *Letting Through
Light* (Ferns and Dutt 1999). But I believe it is essential that
training is seen as a part of institutional changes in general and not
as something in isolation from the rest of what goes on in an
institution. And, even more importantly, I believe that what one
can expect from such training under the present circumstances is
very limited indeed.

Over the past twenty years I have been involved in training many
different professional groups involved in mental health work,
including of course trainee psychiatrists. The problem that I (and
others working in this field) encounter is immense. Today, mental
health professionals are trained most of the time in a way that
reflects traditional western psychiatry and mental health practice
incorporating many of the approaches I have criticised throughout
this book. Race and culture training, when available, is usually

added on as something marginal and, by implication, unimportant. In such a context, trainers who provide something very different, or who try to do so, are swimming against the tide. More often than not they are swimming against an even stronger current that is driving the trainees in a very different direction. I believe that training in the present circumstances can, at best, do no more than raise doubts in the minds of those being trained about the authenticity of the practices that they are being taught, occasionally providing them with a glimpse of what a good multicultural mental health service may be like. At worst, such training absolves the institution providing the training from doing much about the problems involved, occasionally even inducing a complacency in those being trained that the training renders them 'culturally competent' to work with all ethnic groups.

Introduction

The message of this book is that changes in psychiatry and mental health services are needed: changes in clinical practice in the statutory, voluntary (not-for-profit) and private sectors, changes in the research field and changes in the training of mental health professionals, especially psychiatrists and psychologists. In the case of service provision in the statutory sector, it is not a matter of finding a 'good practice model' and replicating this but more one of plugging away, perhaps blasting away occasionally, on many fronts, almost irrespective of the overall practice model. Certainly there have been services in Britain (referred to in Chapter 2) that seem likely to have been successful with respect to black and Asian service-user satisfaction. One example is the community project called MOST in south London (Moodley 1995). But others with very different approaches – such as the Home Treatment in north Birmingham (Harding 1995) and the much earlier Transcultural Unit at Bradford (Rack 1982) – have good reputations too as satisfying needs of black and Asian service users. It is likely that good practice in these services were/are more to do with the leadership, dedication and anti-racist approach of members of staff in the projects, rather than the models used in the services themselves. In my view one must be highly suspicious at the time of writing of any suggestion that any one service model is better for black and Asian people than another. What seems to makes the difference is the 'content' of the service in terms of the people working within it, their attitudes and understanding and ability to work with, rather than against, users of services, together with firmly implemented policies and procedures that address racism. That is the micro-picture of service provision. But this book is more concerned with the larger picture – how services as a whole can be changed for the better so that the changes last into the future.

In Chapter 2 I referred to possible changes in the training of psychiatrists. Clearly, if psychiatric and psychological training can produce psychiatrists and psychologists who are culturally sensitive and trained or induced to be anti-racist, all the better. But that by itself is not going to lead to significant, lasting changes in the practice of psychiatry and psychology because of the fundamental issues within these disciplines. It is only when these disciplines themselves are relevant and appropriate for a modern multicultural society that training can be developed to reflect what is needed. The practitioners of this modernised psychiatry and psychology would then be in a position to do the training. Until then, changes will necessarily be superficial, hopefully a little better than purely cosmetic. But that is better than nothing.

Moving forward means changing psychiatry as a system, especially since psychiatry, as an institution and body of (what goes for) knowledge, has a powerful effect on society in general. However, the quality of service provision is not just dependent on psychiatrists. The management of statutory mental health services too needs to change. In my view, it is far too often the case that managers are more concerned with paper policies than with service quality, as evident by the experience of service users. In other words, systemic changes are required. And, of course, changes must be reflected in changes in the legal framework within which mental health care is provided.

There have been many community projects in the voluntary sector serving black and Asian people and many of these have not been written up or publicised, although they are often greatly appreciated by those who use the services. And here too, as in statutory services, there is no single model that one can identify as being clearly better than another for black or Asian people. The lesson to draw from experience in this sector is the need for variety and the need for special (ethnic-specific) projects that are closely linked to black communities, so that black and Asian people can easily identify with them. In my view there is a need for these to be led by people from the communities that they aim to serve, and it is generally preferable that the majority of therapists employed in such services are from these communities.

Finally, there is a need to consider forensic psychiatry services as a separate issue. I believe that racism in psychiatric practice is the main problem here and something that society as a whole needs to tackle directly. I am not addressing the specific questions around forensic psychiatry in this book because the jointly authored book *Forensic Psychiatry, Race and Culture* (Fernando *et al.* 1998) has explored these fully and proposed possible remedies that can be implemented. But clearly in the long run it is about changing the practice of psychiatry, its inappropriate and oppressive diagnostic practices, risk assessments, and so on. And here too it is not just a matter of changing attitudes among psychiatrists alone, or even a matter of attitude change in general. It is about *systemic* change, challenging deeply rooted vested interests.

Strategies for change

In devising strategies for moving forward, first there is the question of improving the practice of psychiatry. In an earlier book (Fernando 1995d) I postulated a move towards a multisystemic basis for evaluating mental health problems. In another book (Fernando 1991, 2002) I explored ways of combining and using technologies from various cultural sources for a psychiatry that is universally applicable. Both of these sets of ideas still stand but I now realise that the fundamental changes that they imply may not be politically feasible yet, given the state of power politics in the world today – and in psychiatry. However, we can, I believe, move towards a more just and fair system of psychiatric practice by instituting relatively minor changes in the first place. In Chapter 3, I argue that the system of diagnosing mental illness, the psychiatric system, places an enormous emphasis on making judgements about behaviour, thinking and feelings in terms of whether these are right or wrong. That is the basis of diagnosis and the basis of the power of psychiatry. And allied to this power is the stigma associated with many psychiatric diagnoses – psychiatric stigma. Also in Chapter 3 I show that the concept of psychosis is fundamental to the philosophy of psychiatry; and I note that there is a tendency today in Britain to use the term psychosis as being synonymous with schizophrenia. Then, in Chapter 4, I show that racism has become bound up with the schizophrenia diagnosis and hence the stigma carried by it. Institutional racism works through diagnosis because diagnosis is based on judgements that represent ways of thinking about the human condition. The diagnosis of either schizophrenia or psychosis has become both stigmatising and racist. So, as the schizophrenia diagnosis and racism feed on each other in a symbiotic relationship, any attempt to shift racism in psychiatry is resisted because it disturbs the diagnostic model that is seen as important for psychiatry.

In the first section of this chapter I consider strategies for moving psychiatry away from its dependence on diagnosis, especially the diagnosis of schizophrenia. Another allied topic is the issue of paranoia discussed in Chapter 3. Its place as a part of the concept of schizophrenia has never been very stable in psychiatric thinking. I think it is now time to move on, in the light of arguments that I present in Chapter 3. I then indicate in this chapter the importance of understanding the realities of life for black and Asian people in a racist society and the strategies used by them to counteract the effects of racism on the individual. There is little doubt that medication does help some people in trouble, but why it does so is far from clear. What *is* clear is that psychotropic medications are not *curing* any specific illness, although they may help people to cope with mental health problems by suppressing the intensity of feelings that cause problems – or even eradicating them. So I suggest a model within which medication can be used in a humane and helpful way.

Psychiatric therapies are not limited by theoretical constraints because mostly they have always been pragmatic. So psychiatry can, if it only stretches out beyond its narrow horizons of medication, include a diversity of approaches derived from various cultural traditions. So moving forward means addressing the fact that various diverse approaches may be subsumed under the umbrella of 'therapy'. These may involve what may be seen as religious ceremonies or culturally patterned ways of communication; palmistry, fortune telling and astrology too could be included here, possibly being combined with 'talking' in a western tradition. Changes within the discipline of psychiatry must be accompanied by strategies to promote changes in training, and also by other wider strategies that have an effect on the whole mental health system. Training of all professional staff is important but this training must be within a policy that promotes racial equality and it must be applied consistently and effectively. Thus, I have a section on institutional change; this is far from comprehensive but provides an outline for what is needed and possible.

Mental health services are not just those provided in the statutory sector. As we have seen in Chapter 2, the black voluntary sector plays a significant role in supporting black and Asian clients suffering from mental health problems. Many projects in the voluntary sector focus on counselling and psychotherapy. They have made little headway in redressing the injustices in mainstream psychiatry and most people, white and black, have to access these mainstream services in times of need whether they like it or not. In particular the black voluntary sector has a very marginal effect, if any effect at all, in the case of people who get 'sectioned' (compulsorily admitted to hospital), especially those who end up in the hands of forensic psychiatry. Therefore, I suggest in this chapter that the black voluntary sector should be strengthened.

The gamut of therapies subsumed under the terms psychotherapy and counselling – usually referred to as 'talking therapies' – are often looked to as an alternative to traditional psychiatry by people who find the latter unhelpful or even oppressive. The way forward in this field is even more difficult to envisage than it is in the case of ordinary psychiatry. The training in and practice of psychotherapy and counselling, in most settings, are closely tied up with western culture and world views inherent therein. Also, racism is subtly, but very deeply, embedded in psychological theories that underpin the practice of psychotherapy and counselling. So, psychotherapy and counselling need to be revised and perhaps remodelled.

There are many ways in which black and minority ethnic communities are blocked from accessing services. Of course enabling access to all sections of society according to need must go hand in hand with improving the suitability of services to all sections of the community. But there are specific ways in which barriers to service access can be taken down or circumvented. The failure of many services to address the diversity of languages used by the people they are supposed to serve is an obvious barrier to access. But this is only the tip of an iceberg of issues around communication. The language used by psychiatry and psychology often fails to make any sense to the people using mental health services. Being told that one 'has schizophrenia' or 'suffers from depression' interpreted as a biological illness seldom has any meaning when the people concerned know fully well that they have problems that need exploring, relationships that are at fault, and situations that upset them. And then to decry any reference to spiritual aspects of human life, to religion or the supernatural – and even worse attributing such ideas to pathological thinking that denotes illness – is a major barrier between psychiatry and the perceptions of ordinary people.

Finally, there is the vexed question of psychiatric research. Surely if, after a hundred years of researching schizophrenia as an illness, we have got nowhere the message is clear. But there is much more reason than that to re-appraise the psychiatric research agenda. There is far too much money spent on ivory-tower research. Again, vested interests have to be challenged if the research agenda is to change, but change it must if the struggle against racism and for multiculturalism is to move forward. All the strategies for change that I address in this chapter – in psychiatry, in institutional practices, in strengthening the voluntary sector, in counselling and psychotherapy, in access to services, and in psychiatric research – need to be seen in context. I look at these matters in the context of British society and the British version of a multicultural society. Clearly, strategies for change in other places, for example in German or North American society, may be different. Yet some of what I propose here may be universally valid, in particular my comments about changes in diagnostic style and the use of medication.

Revising psychiatric practice

I aim here to pinpoint some areas in which change could occur without too much upheaval. Doing something about the diagnosis of schizophrenia is the first. I believe that unless and until this diagnosis is sufficiently destabilised for it to lose its power both within psychiatry and in the general knowledge of society, the struggle against racism in psychiatry will be stymied. So, any strategy to shift racism in mental health services must find some way of removing schizophrenia from its dominating role. Hopefully, once this is done it will eventually disappear completely from the psychiatric toolbox. Any national strategy for addressing racism in mental health services should be measured against the seriousness with which it addresses this matter. Allied to some progress with the problem of schizophrenia is the issue of paranoia. Both these issues are related to developing ways of taking account of the black experience in society. Finally, I believe that a pragmatic use of medication and the widening of what is meant by psychiatric treatment are feasible. All these ideas and suggestions are not presented as solutions to the current problems of race and culture but as ways of shifting psychiatric practice into a new era. I believe that all these changes are achievable here and now. They are not dependent on radical changes but do require a will to bring about change.

What to do about schizophrenia

The case for abandoning schizophrenia as a diagnosis was presented in Chapter 4. The general push is clear but the resistance is also strong, especially in mainstream psychiatry. Charlton (2000) refers to researchers being 'locked into the present system by a vast infrastructure of journals, conferences and books that are wholly or partially devoted to schizophrenia research' (2000: 138), but he points out (rightly in my opinion) that the main block within the psychiatric profession to dropping the schizophrenia diagnosis is that 'schizophrenia is at the very heart of psychiatry both as a profession and as a research enterprise because it is the classic form of madness' (2000: 139). Marshall believes that 'mainstream psychiatry, particularly in Britain, has established such a rigorous party line that anything questioning the dominant beliefs [about schizophrenia] is likely to be rejected for publication, and denigrated in shrill fashion when appearing in presses outside its control' (1995: 55). Indeed, anyone reading psychiatric journals is bombarded with papers about schizophrenia, peer reviewed papers at that, in which the validity of the concept of schizophrenia is not questioned at all, although, scientifically speaking, such questioning should be insisted upon by the editors of the journals. When, in 1996, I wrote to the editor of the *British Journal of Psychiatry* questioning the validity and usefulness of diagnosing psychosis in black people in Britain, my letter was rejected for publication because (as stated by the correspondence editor of the journal) 'the points made would be familiar to most researchers and readers' (Personal Communication 1996). A disingenuous argument if ever there was one.

However, it is not just blind belief in schizophrenia by psychiatrists that is the problem. I believe that the interlinking of schizophrenia with the social and political systems of western countries – and increasingly those of the non-western world too – have rendered the barriers to it being abandoned even more powerful. Foucault (1988) points out that the use of psychiatry for repressive purposes came about in the Soviet Union when there was a need to 'find a replacement for Stalinism' (1988: 179). During the reign of Stalin, political dissidents were exiled to the gulags in Siberia, but when 'liberalisation' of the political system took place under Khrushchev in the 1960s psychiatry was used for incarcerating political dissidents as described by Bloch and Reddaway (1984). Thus, schizophrenia, and indeed any psychiatric diagnosis, is more likely to be used for political purposes unwittingly or deliberately within a liberal, democratic system than it is in a totalitarian system. In my view, schizophrenia and psychosis have become integrated with the social control exercised by western states both directly and (even more importantly) indirectly. And since racism is a hidden part of the way schizophrenia is diagnosed and perpetuated, the existence of the diagnosis draws psychiatry into the racist control of black people.

One of the early and most persistent critics of schizophrenia, Richard Bentall (1990), suggests deconstructing schizophrenia into its symptoms (such as hallucinations, delusions, 'negative symptoms') and then 'taking the symptoms at face value' (1990: 50) in order to study their cognitive, neurobiological and other correlates. In his book *The Suspended Revolution*, David Healy (1990a), a psychiatrist, points out the limitations inherent in seeing schizophrenia as an illness and advocates a symptomatic approach to the understanding and treatment of the symptoms of schizophrenia. Another psychiatrist, Philip Thomas (1997), suggests that 'we move away from the use of "schizophrenia" as a diagnostic entity and study symptoms in their own right' (1997: 102). And Bruce Charlton (2000) believes that 'the diagnosis tells you less than the symptoms about the best focus for therapeutic intervention' (2000: 137). In my view, moving towards a symptomatic approach and discounting schizophrenia as a diagnosis would be a step in the right direction, but only a small step. Looked at from a transcultural and anti-racist perspective, dismantling schizophrenia into symptoms is not enough, unless it leads on to ways of working in psychiatry that result in the problems represented within schizophrenia being seen outside a strictly medical framework of illness. In other words, these problems must then be opened up to be seen in social, political and cultural contexts.

First and foremost, what are regarded as symptoms must be rendered culture sensitive; they must be seen primarily as individual experiences to be explored in a socio-cultural context for their meaning and significance. Further, the analysis of behaviours, feelings or beliefs as symptoms must be made in the context of social pressures (connected with housing, racism, etc.) impinging on people supposed to have these symptoms and the effect of stereotypes carried in society about them. The preconceptions (in terms of historic attitudes about illness and stereotypes of people who are schizophrenic) held by professionals who make diagnoses, or preconceptions held by others that feed into the making of psychiatric assessments, must be excluded. Finally, the effect on the people assessed by psychiatrists and psychologists must be taken on board through their views expressed directly and through advocates and carers. In other words, identifying symptoms must be a transparent and joint exercise between professionals responsible for making the diagnosis and the person who is being diagnosed, together with his or her advocate and (if appropriate) carer.

Moving from schizophrenia as an overarching diagnosis into a symptomatic approach that identifies, or attempts to identify, symptoms, introducing the sort of modifications to the process of identifying symptoms that I have suggested above, ties in with the current changes in community care arrangements envisaged in the National Service Framework (Department of Health 1999). This framework makes the point that 'black and minority ethnic communities [currently] lack confidence in mental health services . . . [and] services must be planned and implemented in partnership with local communities, and involve service users and carers' (1999: 17). The framework makes it clear that 'specific arrangements should be in place to ensure: service user and carer involvement, advocacy arrangements, integration of care management and the Care Programme Approach (CPA) [and] effective partnerships with primary health care, social services, housing and other agencies including where appropriate, the independent sector' (1999: 10). A reasonable approach within these aims would be for the Department of Health to set down a strategy for enabling the dismantling of schizophrenia in the way I have suggested. Then guidelines can be drawn up within which psychiatrists and others can implement the changes to their practice; professional organisations (such as the Royal College of Psychiatrists) and service users groups would be involved in drawing these up.

Designating 'paranoia' as a 'neurotic' problem

In Chapter 3 I discuss two inter-related matters that apply to the diagnosis of paranoid schizophrenia. First, I argue (in the section 'Holistic thinking') that many people from non-western cultural backgrounds tend to think in a style that connects together (as it were) experiences and feelings about experiences; and that they feel, believe and know rather than *have* feelings, *hold* beliefs and *possess* knowledge. This way of thinking contrasts with a way of thinking that experiences events as separate episodes unconnected with feelings (where inter-connections between such episodes are non-existent unless proven otherwise) and distinguishes objectified feelings, objectified beliefs and objectified knowledge as 'things' in separate compartments as it were. I point to mistakes that may arise if this difference in thinking style is not appreciated, resulting in misidentification of thinking as being 'paranoid'. The second matter concerns the problem inherent in diagnosing paranoid schizophrenia when the only symptom is paranoia, especially when the diagnosis is given to black people living in a racist society. This was commented upon under 'False and true beliefs' in Chapter 3. I argue, following Charlton's thesis, that beliefs identified within the syndrome designated 'paranoia' or 'delusional disorder' as symptoms are 'theory of mind delusions' and not 'bizarre delusions' (Charlton 2000: 39, 43). Basically, such instances are problems of attribution – the fact that the person concerned has attributed certain dispositions, motivations and intentions to a person or group of persons.

Finally, there is the issue of diversity in emotional expression and/or the expression of distress tied up with differences in ways of coping with stress. I discuss this topic at some length elsewhere (Fernando 2002: 60–6). I argue there that culture plays a large part in the way people deal with stress and interpret their feelings. But, in addition, life experience plays a part too. People who are constantly being harassed by society for no fault of their own are much more likely to attribute individual failures or felt stresses to social inequality seen as the fault of other people than to their own personal fault. The result of this is that their coping strategy to deal with anxiety (fashioned by life experience) is to project their feelings, i.e. blame other people for their suffering. A recent study in the US (Friedman and Paradis 2002) highlights the likelihood that African Americans and African-Caribbean immigrants to the

US express anxiety differently to the way in which it is usually assumed as being expressed in psychiatric and psychological 'knowledge'. The researchers concerned point to their finding of a 'diagnostic bias' when people from these groups (essentially black people) are seen in inner-city out-patient clinics: instead of being given a diagnosis of panic disorder (severe anxiety), they tend to be diagnosed as suffering from 'severe pathology' such as 'adjustment disorder with psychosis' or 'schizophrenia' (2002: 182–3). The researchers found that, unlike white Americans, black clients expressed anxiety through 'fears of dying and going crazy' but also attributed symptoms caused by anxiety, such as 'sleep paralysis' (a sensation of being paralysed), 'in the context of their spiritual and cultural beliefs' to causes such as being 'a special target of evil forces' (2002: 184–6). In other words, anxiety was expressed in terms of what may well be called paranoia and misinterpreted as being caused by psychosis or schizophrenia.

In my view, holistic thinking should be recognised and allowed for very specifically. This would result in a significant fall in the identification of paranoia among black people. Second, when erroneous attribution is the problem, the issue should not be seen as a problem (or symptom) of madness (or psychosis/schizophrenia). The problem lies in the way the person has related to others in a particular context – a way that may be maladaptive but as much to do with other people as it is with the person concerned. Paranoia without any disturbance of consciousness should be seen as a problem not a symptom of illness. Then it could be seen as a mental health problem similar to, say, obsessions or a problem of personality or relationships. From that, the approach would be to look for the underlying anxiety causing the paranoia, bearing in mind that culture and life experience play a part in the way anxiety is felt and expressed. In other words, paranoia as a problem should be seen as something neurotic rather than psychotic. Although at times suppressing anxiety or unwanted or intrusive feelings (e.g. by tranquillisers) may be helpful, a constructive approach to therapy is to work through the feelings or beliefs in psychotherapy. I believe that the change I have described in the approach to paranoia is a step towards unravelling racism in the mental illness category that is now diagnosed as delusional disorder (and often as paranoid schizophrenia).

My personal experience in dealing with black and Asian people diagnosed as having paranoid delusions or being paranoid or showing paranoia, has taught me that careful evaluation is required as to the nature of what is meant. The premises upon which their apparently false beliefs derive, the attribution styles they use and the ways of thinking (e.g. holistic thinking, see pp. 124–7) need to be considered in a framework that gives precedence to understanding their feelings (of paranoia). Clinically, I find that dealing with so-called delusions as a problem in the way indicated above is much more constructive and reasonable than dealing with them as a part of illness. This approach does not deviate very much from the medical model of psychiatry but will be productive in terms of helping the individual. In statistical terms, such an approach may considerably reduce the over-representation of black people within the schizophrenia category.

The 'black experience' and strategies to counter racism

Racism is pervasive in British society. Most black and Asian people deal with racism by learning strategies to side-step racism and/or to counteract its effects on their psychological and social functioning. This learning may sometimes be covert in that it is something that is absorbed through socialisation in families and communities. Many of these strategies are to do with behaviour when confronted by the police or when approaching people in authority. These are obvious. What are less obvious are the more subtle strategies that black and Asian people learn, or more correctly absorb, over the years as ways of thinking and behaving that eventually come naturally to them. One problem is that when black and Asian people come into contact with the psychiatric system, some of these strategies may be interpreted in psychiatric jargon as symptoms of illness. The results could be disastrous.

Debasing of self-esteem is something that racism, especially when it is subtle, induces. A common strategy to deal with this is an assumed heightened self-importance – an instinctive feeling that one is someone special or comes from a superior culture or family. In a psychiatric context, this may be seen as grandiosity. Another strategy is described by Grier and Cobbs (1969) in the US as 'healthy cultural paranoia' (see p. 131). This is a sort of suspiciousness and/or avoidance of white society, and perhaps people perceived as white in that they represent white society, as a protective measure. But then in a multi-racial society complete avoidance is not feasible and in any case other black people may be perceived as white when they are fulfilling certain roles, especially in positions of authority. In this instance, the psychiatric label that gets attached is likely to be (pathological rather than healthy, and perhaps even psychotic) paranoia or at least a (neurotic) 'chip-on-the-shoulder'. Once a serious individualised problem, or worse an illness, is deemed to be present, the risk is that the true nature of a situation is ignored. And the result may be that black people presenting to psychiatry get dealt with in an oppressive and damaging manner. Then, psychiatry and psychology become a part of their problem rather than a part of systems through which they may get help. The following three vignettes, based on case histories and narratives of real people known to the author but with details and names changed, illustrate some of this.

Joseph was a 36-year-old (black) African-Caribbean man who was apprehended by the police when he attempted to force his attention on an ex-girlfriend. When the police were called, he talked loudly and told them that he was a prince. The police were overtly friendly towards him but tricked him into allowing them to transport him to a mental health unit for admission. When he realised what was happening, he resisted physically and was heavily restrained and later injected with medication. 'Grandiosity' and 'behaviour disturbance' resulted in a diagnosis of hypomania. Once he got over the initial trauma of admission, he talked calmly about his own import-ance. While still a young boy Joseph had been told by his father that 'whatever white people do to you remember that you are of royal ancestry'; and his father gave him an ivory-headed walking stick to prove this background. It is this knowledge that had carried him through many adverse circum-stances, living in a deprived area where black people had once rioted. Joseph believed that he was destined to be an example to black youth in London. Once this man's beliefs were accepted as valid, he agreed to compromise with society by keeping them to himself and to take some medication to keep 'calm' when he got excited under stress. But he required recurrent help and intercession to deal with neighbours who wanted to get him out of the area and the police who ques-tioned him repeatedly.

Shahid was a young man of 17 when he arrived from Bangladesh to join his parents in England. Three months later he was admitted to a psychiatric unit for observation after apparently becoming aggressive and agitated at home. After that he was in and out of hospital for two years with a diagnosis of borderline disorder/schizophrenia and learning difficulties in a context of family stresses. Although 'aggressive' at home, when in hospital he was well behaved but 'grandiose and deluded' in that he claimed to be a doctor, to own other people's belongings, and to be 'in charge' of other patients. At times he was preoccupied, apparently 'listening' to inner voices. After much consideration, it was decided by the mental health team that Shahid's problems should be seen as primarily stemming from family conflicts and removal from home during crises was counterproductive. Therefore, family interviews were begun and admission to hospital was resisted when the next crisis occurred.

When this crisis happened, the family called the police and Shahid was arrested. On release from custody he was found to be injured (probably as a result of being assaulted while in custody) and so the earlier decision to resist admission to hospital was reversed. He then became 'stuck' in hospital because discharge invariably led to conflict with his family. He continued to be 'grandiose and deluded' in hospital, improving on a small dose of medication but 'relapsing' whenever discharge was considered. This pattern, together with Shahid's apparent difficulty in facing up to the reality of his situation, led to confirmation that he was chronically 'psychotic'. After many months and several failed trials in a variety of community placements, Shahid finally achieved some stability in a hostel with Bangladeshi staff, but continued to require a small dose of a major tranquilliser.

Sharon was a 30-year-old black woman who was admitted to a psychiatric unit after she set fire to some furniture in her flat. She was extremely suspicious of people in the unit and was convinced that people around her wanted to put her down. She claimed to be 'better' than everyone else and that she had been prevented from achieving much by the manipulations of people 'out there'. She denied experiencing hallucinations but appeared to respond to inner voices. During the next two years, she was in and out of hospital and under 'community care' in between admissions. Much of her anger and open hostility was less evident while on a major tranquilliser. The diagnosis of paranoid schizophrenia was made repeatedly.

In the course of discussions with therapists and counsellors Sharon talked about her anger towards her (black) parents for 'pretending to be white', living in a middle-class white area and denying the existence of racism. She had been bullied at school where she was the only black pupil in her class. During most of her teenage years, she had felt that people on the street watched her movements. After leaving school she lived in an area with a large black population but people there shunned her and so she moved back to live near her parents. She felt an urge to destroy whatever she identified as property owned by white society.

After several admissions to an open psychiatric unit, where at times she was deemed 'unmanageable', Sharon was transferred to a secure (forensic) hospital far away from her home town. There she apparently learned 'to play the system' (at least that is how she saw her 'progress') and when discharged she decided to live in a town near that hospital, far away from her parents and the 'white society' of the city that she had grown up in. Her contact with psychiatric services then ceased.

The brief vignettes described above represent people who were struggling with racism, using strategies that were misconstrued by the psychiatric system as paranoia and grandiosity. Major mental illness was diagnosed in each instance and apparent suppression of overt pathological behaviour interpreted as response to treatment with medication. The reality of pressures from society, often represented by police, both added to their problems and undermined efforts to help them deal with family issues. In all three instances, they were partially rescued through interventions that took them seriously as black people but such interventions have limited use while society itself is hostile.

Using medication pragmatically

As psychiatry functions within a medical model, the general approach is to use medication to treat illnesses. However, the limitations of this narrow illness model in psychiatry are now self-evident and have been discussed in various parts of this book, especially in Chapter 3. The approach in current clinical practice is to assume that the illness has a biological origin and so the first line of treatment tends to be medication. In this model, psychiatric drugs are supposed to counteract 'abnormal' biochemistry. But no one has shown how medications counteract mental illness or even the symptoms of mental illness. However, there is some indication that most medications suppress or blunt feelings (Healy 1990b; Charlton 2000), in other words they act as tranquillisers. The specificity of this suppressive action is not clear and is something for research. Healy (1990b) states that 'neuroleptics induce a feeling of indifference in the face of stress – an "antiagitation" effect. This they do in anyone who has them, whether schizophrenic or not' (1990b: 37).

If we accept the above argument – and the experience of people who take neuroleptics tends to support it – it is possible that feelings may be suppressed differentially depending on the person or circumstances, or indeed some neuroleptic drugs may block angry feelings, others attenuate depressive feelings and still others relieve feelings of frustration, or feelings that cannot easily be put into words such as those that come to us as 'voices' talking to us. People who benefit from taking neuroleptics may have to find out exactly how the drugs affect them; how the 'benefit' works for the individual. So, it is their reports that must guide its use and one person's experience may be different from another's. Many people who take psychotropic (neuroleptic) medication tell me that when they do they feel 'detached' or 'distanced' from strong feelings. So, in the case of some people at least, suppression may not be the correct word. I believe that this approach to the use of psychotropic medication can be pursued in practice – an approach that is disengaged from diagnosis. Clearly, research into the subjective feelings of people who use medication is required.

Thus, I believe that psychotropic drugs can be used pragmatically, being guided by the subjective experiences of people who use them. It may sometimes be a good thing to suppress feelings because they are very disturbing or clearly felt as alien to one's existence. Also, it may be necessary to suppress feelings in order to enable a person to get on with her or his life, while seeking ways of understanding the reasons for feeling the way they feel. But sometimes suppressing feelings may *not* be so good for some people. Few people would want to suppress feelings of affection for people close to them. Feelings that enable a person to feel continuity with people whom they love but have died may be valuable feelings to maintain. But the situation may be more complex. Suppressing anger that is justified, say anger about racism, may just mean that the person becomes a doormat for others to tread on. Or suppressing feelings too strongly may result in a person becoming a 'vegetable', a 'zombie' who cannot look after themselves properly. In my view, medication can be used imaginatively and constructively once it is detached from diagnosis. But it would be a matter of balancing the pros and cons – balancing the 'good' that it may do against its 'bad' effects. And mostly, the user of a mental health service, together with the carer, is the best judge of this.

Widening the scope of psychiatric treatment

In the present day psychiatric treatment focuses almost entirely on physical (as opposed to psychological) medical-type therapies, medication and electroplexy (ECT) being the main ones. Other ways of helping people, such as counselling, psychotherapy, social support, etc., are seen as marginal to the main therapeutic programme. However, it was not always like that; for example, the crisis intervention movement and the therapeutic community movement of the 1960s and 1970s (Chapter 3) emphasised social networks and family support as the basis of therapy. Even today, systemic approaches of family therapy (see Minuchin and Fishman 1981) and some psychological therapies (see Haley 1963) tend not to be based on a purely illness approach to mental problems, although most therapists using these approaches still adhere to the basic diagnostic medical model of psychiatry in selecting or accepting people for therapy, including the implications of this model that, for instance, people with a diagnosis of schizophrenia require medication primarily and seldom benefit from 'talking therapies'. The dogma that psychiatric services adhere to in most places is that psychiatry is a medical discipline, mental illness has a biological basis and treatment is aimed at altering functions of the brain. We need to move beyond this dogma.

In moving forward into an age when psychiatry is truly multicultural, therapies from non-western cultural traditions need to be brought in. The difficulties of using these within a narrow medical model are immense. But some movement may be made by, for example, bringing into the arena of psychiatric therapy 'complementary' or 'alternative' therapies used on a pragmatic basis. The primary issue is one of status since medication and ECT too are largely used pragmatically as there is no known rationale to explain any benefit they have. So, the first requirement is for direction from the professional bodies such as the Royal College of Psychiatrists. The College should state that complementary therapies have a place in the psychiatric world. Then training in these therapies should be offered to psychiatrists and others in the mental health scene, and guidelines for their use set out. It is then only a matter of time before the National Health Service has to provide access to these therapies.

Institutional changes and training

In Chapter 2, I write about the issues that black people have brought up at meetings about mental health. Some of the themes for action that have come up time and time again are shown in Box 5.1. Although changes in training are high on the list, most people accept that they must be instituted in a context where training can be effective in changing practice. In other words, training can only be effective within a structure that pursues institutional change. Also, the point is often made that counteracting racism is not dependent so much on training as on changes in attitude and a determination to face up to racism. In other words, it is more about political will than about training of staff.

A broad outline of the institutional context which is required for changes to take place is given in Box 5.2. It is now a legal duty of all public bodies in Britain to promote equality, to look into their institutional processes and minimise – if not eliminate – racism (see Chapter 2). The Department of Health is supposed to do this and so should all health authorities in the country. Each authority has been asked to produce a Race Equality Strategy of Intent. I believe that the Royal College of Psychiatrists too has devised one. In such a strategy, training is likely to figure prominently. But training alone will never suffice. I know from participating in meetings to discuss race and culture training for psychiatrists in February 2001 (see Chapter 2) that little if any change can be expected from the deliberations of this College. And significantly, black and Asian service users have not been consulted.

Once there are changes in the clinical practice of psychiatry these will necessarily be reflected in changes in the legal framework of practice – the Mental Health Act. I am not considering here possible changes in this legal framework: some suggestions were

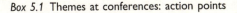

Box 5.1 Themes at conferences: action points

Change professional training and practice
  too eurocentric
  racist attitudes

Counteract racism in services
  institutional racism
  personal prejudice

Counteract discrimination in employment
  tokenism in implementing equal opportunity policies

Forensic psychiatry and 'sectioning'
  racist stereotyping
  cultural insensitivity

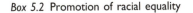

Box 5.2 Promotion of racial equality

Race equality policy
  combating racism
  promoting equal opportunity

Monitoring systems
  employment practices
  service provision
  training
  research

Action at various levels
  disciplinary procedures
  user involvement

Forward planning
  feed in policy, monitoring and action

made in an earlier book (Fernando *et al.* 1998). The point I make is that, in my view, the changes in psychiatric practice must come first. Admittedly, the legal changes currently (at the time of writing) proposed by the British government (Department of Health 2002), with a wide definition of mental disorder and legalisation of compulsory treatment outside hospital, would (if carried into legislation) result in added difficulties for implementing the sort of

Box 5.3 Aims of training in race and culture

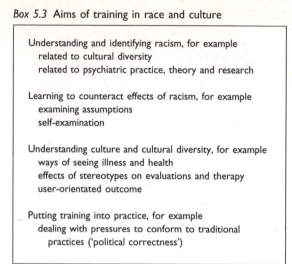

Understanding and identifying racism, for example
   related to cultural diversity
   related to psychiatric practice, theory and research

Learning to counteract effects of racism, for example
   examining assumptions
   self-examination

Understanding culture and cultural diversity, for example
   ways of seeing illness and health
   effects of stereotypes on evaluations and therapy
   user-orientated outcome

Putting training into practice, for example
   dealing with pressures to conform to traditional
     practices ('political correctness')

changes in clinical practice that I suggest here. Yet, if this happens, the changes I propose will be even more necessary. In other words, my view is that, if there is a determination and political will to change professional practice in psychiatry in the way I suggest, the legal framework for the practice of psychiatry cannot by itself stand in the way. Indeed, professionals, especially psychiatrists, may have to work harder and more imaginatively but that is all. Some compromises may have to be made since psychiatry will continue to be expected to implement some degree of social control (in the way it has always done). Certain eventualities may have to be defined for compulsory admission and/or compulsory treatment – perhaps the presence of certain beliefs accompanied by risk of danger, or a certain degree of disturbance of contact with reality, or a level of depression that entails risk to life. But a changed approach in psychiatric practice will undoubtedly result in changes at grass roots for users of services, and that is what is important.

Box 5.3 indicates a basis for a good training scheme but I am not taking the topic of training any further in this book except to make the point that, in this day and age, service users must be actively involved in drawing up training schemes and participating in training of professionals. I believe that a combination of black and Asian service users working with (what one may call) a sort of culture-sensitive anti-racist critical psychiatry and psychology should be the basis of race and culture training in the future. And training is required for workers in both the statutory and voluntary sectors. I reiterate here my view that 'added-on' training in race and culture has a very limited benefit; it is the traditional, mainline, training that has to change and that is only possible once changes have been made in the practice of psychiatry and psychology.

Strengthening the black voluntary sector

The impediments under which the black (including the Asian) voluntary sector functions and the inherent weaknesses within many black voluntary projects are described in Chapter 2. I have heard it stated quite often that applications for grants by black and Asian applicants hoping to extend or set up mental health projects in the voluntary sector are 'poor' – usually meaning that they are not written in a form that adheres to the expectations of traditional grant-giving organisations and fall down when judged on traditional criteria. The interpretation is often that black and Asian projects lack leadership and that the people in charge require training in how to write applications and how to run their projects, or that communication with them is not easy.

In my view, what is quoted as a 'lack of leadership' obscures the basic issue that many funders look for leaders among black and Asian people in the voluntary sector who are like the professionals in the white statutory sector. If leaders are seen as having 'peculiar views' or being outside 'mainstream' they do not even get a look in. Communication problems often obscure issues about trust and understanding. Issues around communication cover much that may be interpreted as rigidity of funding organisations – or downright racism. It is certainly the experience of many black and Asian voluntary sector workers that their applications for funding (in contrast to applications by white people and organisations) are rejected on spurious grounds in many instances. Grant-giving bodies need to address the cultural diversity of what projects (in the black voluntary sector) are about, the variety of interpretations of the meaning of mental health and disorder and the fact that black and Asian people applying for grants may not wish to compromise too much in adhering to established formulae for describing what they wish to do. As in other parts of society traditional systems have to address the fact that society is now multicultural.

I recall being involved several years ago with an Asian group applying for a grant to extend work that they had until then being carrying out unpaid. The voluntary workers had been interceding with local housing officers and hospital professionals on behalf of Asian women who were under pressure in the community. The unpaid workers had gradually reached a point at which they were being called upon for help by social workers, housing officers, psychiatrists and others, ostensibly as interpreters, but clearly as people to support these stressed women. Temporary funding to provide travel expenses was provided while the group applied for funding for their work as a mental health project. Their application was an appropriate one (in my opinion) because the project was directed at women who could (in psychiatric terms) be diagnosed as 'depressed'. The applicants did not view their clients as 'mentally ill' and so I wrote a letter of support pointing out the cultural context in which the work was being carried out. However the grant-giving body rejected the application as being outside their remit because their funds were assigned for 'mental health' projects and not for 'welfare' projects.

There have been several attempts in the past to deal with some of the problems of the black voluntary sector but without any lasting effect. The approach in the past has been to set up a support agency of sorts financed indirectly through government funding, usually by a local authority. I have had some experience of dealing with such an agency in a west London borough when a black voluntary organisation that I was involved in was referred to it by the funders. It was quite evident to me, and to others involved in the black voluntary organisation, that the support agency was lacking in expertise and grossly understaffed. They were clearly unable to advise the voluntary group with their organisational problems, except to load them with references to books and publications. But more than that, the people in charge of the support agency were obviously working hand-in-glove with the funders, who made it very clear that they wanted to close the black project in spite of evidence from users of their service that it was highly thought of. It is not an uncommon experience of black voluntary groups that the support agencies that they are referred to are inadequate and are often in collusion with funders. Agencies to support the black voluntary sector on a countrywide basis, that are not tied to funders, have been established in the past but have not lasted for long. The reasons for their failure are not clear but I believe that they are similar to those outlined in Chapter 2 as problems affecting the black voluntary sector generally. In my opinion, a careful analysis of past attempts at setting up umbrella organisations to support the black voluntary sector is required before any further top-down attempts are made on this line.

I believe that supporting the black voluntary sector is crucial for the struggle against racism in psychiatry and mental health services. In my view, it is necessary to encourage and promote a bottom-up approach to this problem. A possible way forward is to encourage black service users and carers to form an organisation, led by people who have their confidence to start with. Perhaps something like a national black alliance for improvement of mental health services may be a possible outcome. Such a body has to be entirely separate from white organisations. The way that the service user group 'Survivors Speak Out' was formed and supported may be a model to follow in some respects. However, I believe that there are significant differences between the 'black scene' and the 'white scene' in the mental health field. In exploring the user/survivor movement in relation to black and Asian people, Sassoon and Lindow (1995) write

> Both groups [black and Asian] have not, on the whole, been involved in the movement's campaigning aspects. The fact that they are less involved implies that the philosophy of empowerment in some respects may have been constructed in line with dominant white values and that many black users may prefer alternative routes to making their voices heard.
>
> (1995: 89)

Both authors of the book chapter quoted above – one black and one white – have been involved in the service-user movement for many years. Although accepting the importance of user involvement in reforming the psychiatric system through models imported from The Netherlands such as Patients Councils and the Hearing Voices Network, they point out that these models have not been successful in addressing the main problems that black and Asian people face in the mental health system. Moreover, black and Asian service users have on the whole steered clear of these white organisations. Mina Sassoon and Viv Lindow see a need for black people to form their own user movement and suggest that black users and professionals may well work together in such movements (unlike in the white mental health scene), at least up to a point. My experience too suggests that the tendency is for black service users to work in conjunction with some carers and some black professionals, much more so than is the case with white service users. Perhaps a body that brings together black service users, carers and professionals may be a first step towards this aim. It is imperative that such a body should be aware of the power of established vested interests that may seek to undermine it and equally imperative that it should derive its impetus from grass-roots black people.

As stated earlier, the injustices in mainstream psychiatry suffered by black people have hardly been touched in the course of the good work done by the black voluntary sector. The lack of a well-organised black user movement makes it difficult to make progress in this field, but there is the need I believe for active work by health authorities, trusts and professional bodies to take direct action. Much of this book is concerned with the issues that need tackling. I believe that the black voluntary sector can play an important part in this.

The problems of the black voluntary sector (referred to in Chapter 2 and expanded further above, pp. 193–6) have to be addressed first and foremost, especially the issues about funding. In order to widen its scope, the black voluntary sector needs to have a right of access to black patients and their notes, so long as the patients themselves agree. The details of this, such as the accreditation of certain groups to have this right, would need to be worked out Then, funding would be required to enable these voluntary groups to obtain legal representation for black people who are compulsorily detained and on their books. Second, all patients who are compulsorily detained should have a written statement from the hospital outlining their treatment plans and the reasons for the medication being prescribed. These statements should be available to their legal representatives (who could obtain independent opinions on them). I believe that these two minor steps would break into the currently impenetrable psychiatric system that black people find oppressive. Clearly these steps in themselves would not solve any problems but I believe they would move the struggle forward.

Improving psychotherapy and counselling

As society is multicultural, the therapies available within mental health services in society have to be applicable to suit a diversity of cultural traditions. Western psychotherapy is grounded in a world view and ways of thinking that are specifically western. By this I mean that it is underpinned by certain fundamental cultural assumptions about human nature and the human condition. In discussing the application of western psychotherapies in India, China and Japan, Kakar (1995) takes a rather uncompromising approach to the integration of cultures that may be necessary for a multicultural approach to psychotherapy: 'Together with other value-laden beliefs of the Enlightenment – in individual autonomy and individual worth, in the existence of an objective reality that can be known, in the possibility of real choice – the individualist model of man has pervaded contemporary psychotherapy' (1995: 83). I believe that ways of thinking and world views are very different across cultures. But yet there are common themes – points of reference at which they meet. Even more than that therapists can, and should, be able to appreciate the differences, allow for them and use them constructively.

Psychotherapy and counselling, above all other forms of service provision for people identified as having 'mental health problems', depend on effective relationships being formed between the professional(s) and the client(s). Professionals working in Britain inherit a historical tradition of racism that must affect the nature of this relationship unless positive action is taken by the therapist(s) to counteract its effect. Nineteenth-century ideas of race dominated by racist stereotypes of people encountered in Asian and African colonies and the American continent, have fed into building up racist images of criminality and madness, dangerousness and aggressiveness, underdevelopment and primitive cultures. These ideas have informed the disciplines of psychology and psychiatry within which psychotherapy and counselling have developed (Fernando 1991). Thus, racist stereotypes and preconceptions would go into judgements and assumptions that underlie assessments and diagnoses made by psychiatrists, psychologists, psychotherapists and counsellors, unless specific anti-racist measures are taken during training and then carried into practice. People being trained in psychotherapy or counselling must learn how to address racism that is likely to affect their practice.

Training

Training in counselling and psychotherapy, like training in many other disciplines, involve the gathering of knowledge, the development of skills and the promotion of certain attitudes that are seen as necessary for good practice. In the next few paragraphs I present some suggestions for a rethinking of training. These suggestions are by no means comprehensive and are presented merely as a basis for such rethinking. As I have pointed out elsewhere (Introduction), I do not claim to be a psychotherapist or counsellor nor do I claim to be particularly knowledgeable about the training of counsellors and psychotherapists.

Psychologies, such as Buddhist psychology (Chapter 3), that originate in non-western traditions are often fundamentally different from western psychology that underpins psychotherapy and counselling. So, counsellors and psychotherapists working in a multicultural society must have some grounding in these non-western psychologies – at least in sufficient depth to enable them to appreciate where their clients are coming from (psychologically speaking). Training in skills of communication is usually an integral part of the training of psychotherapists and counsellors. If they are being trained to work in a multicultural society the emphasis in training must address cultural variations in communication patterns so that the therapists will be able to (a) avoid the pitfalls leading to misunderstandings because of variations in meanings attached to concepts and the therapists' own preconceptions arising from their backgrounds, unwitting racist assumptions, etc. and (b) understand fully the limitations that are inherent in cross-cultural communication. The latter stem from both cultural difference and differences in background, including, for example, the experience of racism.

Many black and Asian people living in western societies have, over the years, developed strategies for dealing with racism. Some people are aware of these and can verbalise them and explain them to their counsellors and psychotherapists, but others are only partially aware (or occasionally totally unaware) of this aspect of adaptation that they have learned. Therefore, all psychotherapists and counsellors working with black and Asian clients must be trained in recognising strategies used by their clients in a western society and if possible be able to guide their clients in using such strategies. Clearly, it is not a matter of learning about strategies in a mechanical fashion but of developing an ability to suss out and tease out (in the course of psychotherapy or counselling sessions) the nature of the strategies being used by individual clients, and then helping the clients to develop them.

Since psychotherapy and counselling are therapies based on communication, which in turn is based on relationships (between the client and the practitioner), the attitudes of psychotherapists and counsellors inevitably play a significant role in the efficacy of their practices. The attitudes usually promoted as necessary for practice in western societies may not all be suitable when there are intercultural situations, and so may need revising. Most psycho-therapists and counsellors are taught to be non-directive, draw firm boundaries between their personal lives and those of the clients, and to be non-judgemental. All these attitudes may need to be altered to some extent in intercultural work. The ways in which they would need modification are too complex for discussion in this section. The point is that these and other attitudes that are promoted as valuable are geared to ways of communicating and relating that are culturally embedded.

Practice

Changes in the training referred to above must of course be reflected in changes in practice. In talking with service users and therapists, I can see where things seem to be going wrong with these disciplines when they are used in a multicultural setting. However, it is not possible to indicate specific, generalisable direc-tions for change in the practice of psychotherapy and counselling. Unlike the case with psychiatry and clinical psychology, many practitioners of counselling and, to a lesser extent, psychotherapy, have examined their practice in some depth in order to increase the cultural sensitivity of their work. The position so far is that change can come from pursuing particular issues *in practice* on various parameters, in various directions and at various points.

Several multi-authored books present a variety of articles by practitioners working in a British context. These include *Trans-cultural Counselling* (Eleftheriadou 1994), *Race, Culture and Counselling* (Lago and Thompson 1996), *Transcultural Counselling in Action* (D'Ardenne and Mahtani 1999), *Counselling in a Multi-cultural Society* (Palmer and Laungani 1999), *Intercultural Therapy* (Kareem and Littlewood 2000) and *Working with Interpreters in*

Mental Health (Tribe and Raval 2003). These books cover practical issues that need to be addressed by psychotherapists and counsellors working in a multicultural setting in a British context, for example communication, assessment, goal setting, the nature of the therapeutic relationship, family structures, supervision of psychotherapists and counsellors, and working with interpreters. They encompass a wealth of information and opinion about practising psychotherapy and counselling in multicultural settings but have certain limitations.

In my estimation, some matters of importance have been largely omitted from the books listed above. In my view, what is important in the therapeutic relationship between client and their counsellor or psychotherapist is dependent on rapport, even more than on communication at the level of talking. Rapport is related to being aware, and not necessarily at a conscious level, of each other's emotional thinking. It is within such a rapport that support, analysis and sensitivity can be established. I believe that there is the need for psychotherapists and counsellors to appreciate the importance of culturally determined ways of thinking. This topic is covered in Chapter 3 under the headings 'Spirituality and mental health' and 'Holistic thinking'. In my view psychotherapists and counsellors need to develop a mindset that enables them to empathise with connectedness (see pp. 125–7), and be able to integrate a feel for spirituality into the models that they use in understanding their clients. These topics (spirituality and connectedness in thinking) are complex and diverse and the reader is referred to Chapter 3 for their discussion. The point I make here is that moving forward in the field of psychotherapy and counselling must address these issues. How this can be done I must leave to people who are trained in psychotherapy and counselling.

Another issue that is inadequately addressed in the books referred to above is the need for psychotherapists and counsellors to be aware of racism and, more importantly, to develop techniques for counteracting racism. The ways in which racism affects the therapeutic relationship and the attitudes of the practitioners are sometimes referred to, but rarely in any depth. Clearly, none of the therapists who present their views make out any specific model of psychotherapy or counselling – although terms such as 'transcultural counselling' and 'intercultural therapy' are used. Anti-racist training is a subject in itself (e.g. Ferns and Madden 1995) and cannot be covered here. The point to make is that if psychotherapists and counsellors want to move forward, they need to develop knowledge and a plethora of skills in this field.

Enabling access to services

A point that I have already made needs to be repeated here. Improving access to services must go hand in hand with improving their appropriateness to all sections of the population. If a service is to be equitably accessible to all ethnic groups, service providers must, first and foremost, have an understanding of the variety of expectations, concepts of mental health and illness, and attitudes to help seeking, in the community at large. Services can then be planned properly to suit all those who need them. As the focus of mental health care in the British National Health Service moves into primary care, Primary Care Trusts need to address these issues from scratch. Surveys of public attitudes to mental health care in the district covered by a Trust must be a starting point. Ensuring that services are not structured so that they block entry to any one group of people means that the diversity of expectations and attitudes must be addressed. The blocks may be something simple like language barriers or, less obvious but equally simple, off-putting attitudes of staff, but in many instances blocks to access are likely to be multiple.

So, preventing blocks to access may mean looking at the provision of interpreters, although it is preferable to have people on the staff with the requisite language skills. (I am not dealing with issues around the use of interpreters in this book.) Ensuring that people who work the services, particularly the front-line staff such as receptionists, are trained to communicate in ways that make everyone feel welcome, respect cultural diversity and so on, may have to be addressed. Of course, identifying exactly what the blocks are to obtaining *appropriate* and acceptable services – acceptable to potential users of the services that is – has to precede the removal of the blocks. It may be that some staff do not refer people from certain backgrounds for talking therapies because of prevailing stereotypes (of who benefits and who does not from services on offer). And stereotyping may well lead to some types of patient (compared to others) being given medication much too quickly or too frequently. And so on. So, differential service provision must be monitored and here ethnic monitoring is important. Unfortunately, ethnic monitoring of services, introduced in 1993, still seems not be carried out properly in many places. Since the focus of mental health care will eventually be within primary care, Primary Care Trusts must accept responsibility for ensuring it is done and that such monitoring informs their policies on commissioning services in the mental health field.

In fostering mental health in communities and people generally, diversity in the understanding of what mental health means must be taken on board. Sudhir Kakar (1984), an Indian psychoanalyst trained in Europe who has written a great deal about the cultural diversity of what is considered as 'pathology', sees mental health as a 'rubric, a label which covers different perspectives and concerns, such as the absence of incapacitating symptoms, integration of psychological functioning, effective conduct of personal and social life, feelings of ethical and spiritual well-being and so on' (1984: 1). But also, there is a need to understand the fact that pressures on people and on communities can have deleterious effects on mental health; and here racism as a pressure in society must be addressed. The pressures arising from racism are sometimes easy to recognise, for example when there is racial harassment or racial attacks. But sometimes the ways in which racism pressurises is less obvious. It may be the alienation when people feel that they do not *belong* or the racism experienced in everyday interactions; for example, racism may be experienced in interactions with colleagues and supervisors in the work place, or it may be the subtle ways in which people are dealt with in shops that matter, or indeed when trying to get an appointment at a GP surgery. These events and experiences – not very important in isolation – add up in the context of negative images one sees on the television or in ordinary news items in the press causing 'pressure'. It is important that the people who provide psychological and psychiatric services should realise the pressure that this sort of 'everyday racism' (Essed 1990) has on people. And of course these pressures can promote formal illness, especially states of depression which can be generated by low self-esteem and a sense of powerlessness.

In the case of attitudes of professional staff, especially those working in psychiatry and psychology, training in race and culture must play a crucial role. But training must be carried out in a context of policies to combat racism and promote equal opportunities, policies that are implemented and monitored. Involvement of service users at various levels – in planning and in clinical work – is an important way forward generally, and not just in combating inequalities arising from racism and cultural diversity. I suggest that, in commissioning mental health services, Primary Care Trusts should consider the following points.

1. Introducing and monitoring policies and training based on a better understanding of racial and cultural issues in the way services are felt by users, and informed by ethnic monitoring.
2. Promoting self-help type ethno-specific projects, even on a small scale, for ethnic minorities. I believe that this will in time give rise to new models of seeing mental health and illness and new approaches to what we call 'therapy'.
3. Working out strategies for altering practices at an individual level by imaginative approaches to questions of diagnosis and care.
4. Undertaking or commissioning imaginative operational social research can play a part in effecting change.

Changing research

My comments in Chapter 1 criticising psychiatric research should not be applied to all research. Mind (the British National Association for Mental Health) has published a booklet (Patel 1999) that is designed to start a discussion on how psychiatric and psychological research may be rendered less insensitive to issues of race and culture. The agenda can move forward from that and it needs to do so. First, there is now an extensive body of theory and research documenting the ways in which race, ethnicity, gender and class – and other dimensions of social difference and value – are causally linked to mental health problems. The problem is that none of this research seems to touch medical psychiatric research. Second, although research in the sense of systematic investigation and study is as essential in the medical mental health field as in any other, it needs to be properly informed socially, politically and ethically as much as medically and biologically. The problems referred to in Chapter 1 mean that research now needs to be properly controlled and directed. This should not be left to psychiatrists with a system to defend, an axe to grind. The system of peer review, whereby applications for funding of research projects and submissions for publication of papers in professional journals are vetted, and sometimes rejected, on the basis of the opinions of other professionals, needs to be revised drastically. Peer review should be replaced by stakeholder review. All research projects and submissions for publication should be considered by committees composed of representatives of people and groups that have an interest in the matters being pursued. Thus, the majority of people on committees that consider psychiatric research should be service users or representatives of community groups that can speak for service users. This model should be applied to ethics committees that consider research applications too. Third, we cannot ignore the fact that publications in psychiatric and psychological journals carry power and influence. So research investigation into race issues must be progressed, but this must be done in a social and political approach. And not just research funding but also publication must be opened up from its current control by vested interests. I present here specific changes in research methodology and the general nature of mental health research.

Psychiatric research

The approach in most current research is to use diagnoses as valid categories for identifying mental health problems assuming that they are universally valid. In fact, in scientific terms, their validity for use in research is highly questionable. In a review of the clinical validity of syndromes recognised in contemporary psychiatric classifications, Kendell (1989) concludes 'Studying populations of schizophrenics or phobics implicitly assumes that schizophrenia and phobic disorders are valid diagnostic categories and I do not believe that we yet have the evidence to justify such an assumption' (1989: 54). In arguing for a dimensional approach to the measurement of symptoms Brugha (2002) states that that 'although dichotomies can make things look easier . . . discarding variance wastefully diminishes statistical power to explain and predict' (2002: 1150–1). I suggest that psychiatric research should now shift from categories to dimensions in measuring symptoms, and further, such measures must always be supplemented by other ways of identifying mental health problems. These must include methods of measuring problems and needs as identified by people who use, or are deemed to need, mental health services. This is especially important in researching ethnic issues. In its *Strategies for Living Project* the Mental Health Foundation in London has initiated research managed and conducted by service users (Nicholls 2001). At present their approaches are designed to supplement traditional research, but there is a great deal that traditional research can learn from methodologies being pursued in this project. The aim of psychiatric research should be to combine with such projects eventually, but as a first step I suggest that basic psychiatric approaches to the measurement of symptoms are changed in the way I have indicated.

Another issue in research into mental health problems is the usual failure in traditional research circles to address the context in which these problems occur. I believe that study of mental health problems (modified in the ways described above) must be balanced by sociopolitical study of the context in which they occur. In any case, the political context in which research is done should be opened up to allow those who use the services to lead the direction of research. The evaluation of mental health problems must be primarily dependent on the experiences of people who are deemed to 'suffer' them. And psychologies drawn from all traditions should be combined into a universally applicable system for understanding mental health and ill health. All these matters need to be addressed in the light of what is practicable in the multicultural, multi-racial, multi-ethnic society that is Britain.

Another feature of psychiatric research into ethnic issues today is that it is mainly top-down research, where experts (usually at centres of excellence) decide what needs to be researched and how it should be done. Involving service users is nearly always marginal to the main thrust of the research and purely tokenistic. Changing the culture of research so that it is bottom-up (i.e. starts with user views and needs identified by people who suffer mental health problems) is likely to threaten vested interests of the psychiatric establishment and so requires a political will to enforce. In my view, what is required is a re-orientation of most research to concentrate on investigating changes in service provision and ways of implementing it. However, I believe that there is a place for traditional-type research carried out primarily by experts with scientific knowledge and skills.

The agenda for psychiatric research carried out by experts needs to move forward into being directed at:

1. Neuropsychological or biological approaches that examine fundamental feelings that are distressing to people and so count as symptoms; these may include some types of hearing voices, seeing visions, loss of appetite and feelings of depression.

2. The use of techniques, such as drug therapies, exercise, talking therapies focusing on what problems if any are alleviated and what are aggravated, from the point of view of people experiencing problems (mental health problems).

But more than all that, I think that research should focus on developing new ways of working in association with service users, developing techniques that focus on what people with mental health problems see as their wants or their needs. There is no doubt in my mind that important insights may be gained in the field of mental health generally by researching people's experiences of the systems of care that are on offer and researching ways of thinking and helping people with mental health problems that are certainly there in all cultural contexts. But to do this, psychiatry and psychology need to get out of their ethnocentric straitjackets, broaden their cultural bases and address racism. But for research to be consumer or user orientated, the organisation around research funding and the vetting of projects have to change; for example, the majority of people on ethnics committees for psychiatric research should be people who have used psychiatric services and they should represent the ethnic diversity of the population.

Summary

This chapter outlines some areas in which changes can be made without too much upheaval. Clearly, the changes suggested here do not constitute a blueprint for change overall. They are piecemeal and to some extent unconnected but if taken up, at least in part, I believe that psychiatric practice and mental health services in general will greatly improve – not just for black and Asian people but for *everyone*. The changes in clinical psychiatric practice that are suggested here do not disturb significantly the medical illness model that psychiatry is wedded to, but shifts its emphasis from objectifying people to treating those who use mental health services as real people, with real lives in a real world with various pressures, including racism. Further, the changes would enable psychiatrists and others working in the mental health field to see themselves as real people too and not just as professionals acting a role. Thus the way would be set, I hope, for collaboration between people who provide psychiatric and mental health services and those who use them. True user participation can result.

I believe that strengthening the black voluntary sector in the way I have envisaged is not the answer to ethnic issues outlined in earlier chapters. But it will promote change all round, not just by enabling innovative projects to develop that are under black and Asian control, thereby encouraging self-help, but by hopefully setting standards for the statutory sector to aim for. Since most projects in the black voluntary sector provide counselling and psychotherapy, it is in these fields that there is most to gain from supporting the black voluntary sector. However, changes in the training of counsellors and psychotherapists and more general changes in the practice of these skills are necessary, and I outline some directions for change. The removal of impediments to access to mental health services – whether these are discriminatory or not – are alluded to in this chapter, but access and appropriateness must go hand in hand. If services are not appropriate then just improving access may merely exacerbate problems. The final section in this chapter deals with the field of psychiatric research. I point out that changes are needed in the research agenda and also in the tools used for psychiatric research, especially in the field of research into what are called 'ethnic issues'.

Chapter 6

Future prospects

There have been remarkable changes in British society over the past fifty years but psychiatry and psychology have failed to keep up. So, although mental health care has shifted from being mainly in large institutions to being based in the community, with corresponding changes in structural aspects and style of mental health service delivery, changes in the content of the service (from the angle of how it is experienced by people who access or confront the services) have been slight. This is partly because the services are underpinned by psychology and psychiatry that are out of kilter with the needs of a multicultural society. Today's society requires mental health services that are backed up by a psychiatry and a psychology that encompass a variety of cultural traditions; psychotherapy and counselling that are sufficiently flexible to address cultural diversity of society; and research methods that are much wider than the traditional narrow medical focus. In short, society needs mental health services that are geared to the needs of all sections of society.

Whereas in the 1970s black people were asking for changes, blaming white society for marginalising them and ignoring their needs, now the mood among black and Asian people is of quiet self-confidence, claiming the right to be part of society – a multiethnic society – and access to services that are appropriate to their needs. And I believe that that is exactly what white people want too. As the struggle against racism developed in the 1980s, black people in Britain felt that they were alone in their struggle, apparently wanting to be accepted by British society. Today the feeling is that the struggle against racism is a common struggle for society as a whole and, in spite of setbacks, one that will continue to be pursued. Unfortunately, extracting adequate responses from statutory services in the mental health field – responses that go beyond funding conferences – has been like extracting the proverbial water from a stone; and in the case of the professional disciplines such as psychiatry and psychology it has been even worse than that. Over the years many strategies for change have been proposed but very little has changed. The Department of Health in Britain has recently produced yet another strategy to meet inadequacies arising from issues of race and culture. At the time of writing, this strategy is about to be issued in draft form for consultation. Some of the lines along which my own thinking has led me are given in earlier chapters of this book, culminating in some suggested strategies for change in the *short term* that are outlined in Chapter 5. In this final chapter I try to look ahead in time.

Achieving multiculturalism, opposing racism

The debate about multiculturalism in Britain today tends to focus on issues of assimilation and integration, often thought of as opposing forces that act on the newcomer (the immigrant) or members of settled minority ethnic communities. For them, assimilation means the loss, to a lesser or greater degree, of individual culture in deference to that of the majority – the 'host community' in the case of immigrants. And integration is about maintaining differences while becoming a part of wider society. Generally speaking, multiculturalism implies integration rather than assimilation, but what is often forgotten is the responsibility of the majority ethnic communities, 'white people', to accept and adjust to cultural plurality if multiculturalism is to succeed. In other words, the choice, and the implications of the choice, apply both ways; to both the majority and the minority cultural groups. Minorities have to feel accepted (not just tolerated) if they are to become integrated. In fact when there is accommodation from both sides, successful multicultural societies develop. It is a lack of accommodation on *both* sides that characterises areas where ethnic tensions prevail, sometimes blowing up into riots such as those in Oldham and Bradford (in the north of England) in 2001 (Chapter 2). At the heart of the problem lies racism. So the struggle against racism and the movement towards multiculturalism must go hand in hand. However, there is one proviso. In countries where political parties or popular movements that actively foster racial hostility have a voice that is listened to, ethnic tensions are artificially contrived and promoted. This has not happened in Britain to any significant extent except that the British National Party (although relatively weak and ineffectual on a national basis) has been partially successful in gaining support in some parts of the UK, for example in a few northern cities (leading to the riots in Bradford and Oldham in 2001 and the election of three British National Party councillors in Burnley). In Britain the problem is more of institutional racism than politically fostered racism, although the latter is always there as a possible threat to social cohesion.

The struggle against racism forms a major subject matter of this book. To envisage a future when racism is no longer a significant problem for society may be a dream. However, I believe that freedom from its main effects in the field of mental health and psychiatry is possible in the foreseeable future. In Chapter 5, I suggest some changes in psychiatric practice that would erode the power of racism in psychiatry. And, if they gather momentum allied, I hope, to psychiatry reclaiming the high moral ground within the western medical tradition that is enunciated in the Hippocratic oath (see Thomas 1997: 214), we can expect a different sort of psychiatric practice. Not just one where, as Thomas (1997) envisages, 'we [psychiatrists] must allow ourselves to be ourselves with others' (1997: 242), but one where psychiatrists and all mental health professionals appreciate fully both their individual prejudices and the institutionalised racism of their practices, so that they make allowances for their failings, their limitations, and their need for constant self-audit.

Psychiatry claims to be a medical speciality and it is likely to remain so for the foreseeable future, but I hope with many modifications. It is in the course of these modifications that I envisage a widening of its cultural base and a breakdown of racism in its practice. However, it is unlikely to be quite so simple. Psychiatry functions in a society that expects psychiatrists, psychologists and other professionals involved in mental health work to deliver certain outcomes. If psychiatrists generally become culturally sensitive, liberal, and anti-racist, they are likely to come into conflict with society. So a clear lead must be given by the professional bodies concerned. Here too we can rightly expect change. My vision, as a psychiatrist, is of, say, a Royal College of Psychiatrists and a British Psychological Society that is allied to users of psychiatric services in lobbying for resources to help people in need, people suffering from mental distress. But for this to happen both these organisations, particularly the former, must recognise the failings of psychiatry and psychology in a multi-cultural society. Tackling its own institutional racism (as the College is trying to do) is only a start and a minor part of what is needed. Reforming the practice of psychiatry and psychology must be the aim. Black and Asian members of the College have a special responsibility to struggle for this change (and in particular not to collude in preventing it) but it is not just their problem.

I have pointed out many times in this book that racism is deeply embedded in British society. Its internalisation affects everyone including black and Asian people themselves. Liberation from internalised racism may not be an easy task for black and Asian people, but it must be done and they must take action towards making this happen. In the field of research in particular, black and Asian professionals – especially psychiatrists – need to be aware of their special position in safeguarding the anti-racist cause. They have to think seriously of strategies to deal with internalised racism, rather than take the easy option of collusion (Chapter 2). Yet separation, opting out of the system, is not the answer either, because that may lead to even more problems – just as segregated living in some parts of the UK has exacerbated racism (see Chapter 2). In the mental health field ethnospecific services, essentially separate services, may be needed for some considerable time because, even if psychiatry and mental health services themselves counteract racism, racism will continue in society at large and black and Asian people would therefore need somewhere they can feel safe.

Another task for black and Asian psychiatrists – and indeed others from minority ethnic communities working in the mental health field – is to address the serious problems within and between these communities. I do not discuss these in this book. They include racism of Asian people against black people (and vice versa), so-called 'black-on-black violence' (Fernando 1998c), pro-motion of 'macho' male images, physical and emotional abuse in families, forced marriages, and suppression of women's rights. When these problems affect black and Asian people, they are problems for the whole of society and it is right that society as a whole is concerned in dealing with them; just as society as a whole must be concerned with football hooliganism and paedophilia that seem to affect mainly white communities. Black and Asian people must also play their part in social integration: a process that involves all communities. So it is right that the struggle against racism is accompanied by promotion of positive attitudes about people seen as culturally or racially different (ethnically different) among black and Asian communities as well as the promotion of such attitudes among white people.

Multicultural psychiatry

If the changes that I suggest in Chapter 5 are taken up and developed, the future practice of psychiatry may look something like the following: Individual beliefs and experiences of people presenting with mental health problems would be taken seriously; for example, they would not be dismissed as being 'just delusions'. Psychiatrists would move away from seeing 'symptoms' such as hallucinations as 'disorders of form' (see Chapter 3), towards seeing them as experiences with meaning and significance. False beliefs would not be taken as mere 'delusions' (i.e. disorders of form) but as feelings and ideas with meaning, and so the premises on which they are based would be explored. The illness model may not disappear, but the symptoms now taken as indicators of underlying pathology, will become a focus for joint discussion between all concerned. What people believe in, hear, think and feel will take centre stage. The 'schizophrenic' would certainly disappear but also, pejorative labels such as 'the voice hearer' or 'the deluded' would go. Instead we would have people who think differently to most people but who have validity and importance as people in their own right. In this system neither illness nor symptoms will have a stigmatising power and racism can then be tackled without the impediment of having to tackle stigma as well. Medication would no longer be the be-all and end-all of psychiatric treatment. Various approaches will be thought through and discussed with the services user and others involved with him or her. And when medication is used the assessment of its usefulness will be largely in the hands of the person who takes it.

I hope that psychiatry may actually move on even further into becoming truly multicultural. Mental health would be seen as something that is culturally centred. By this I mean that the aims in diagnosing and treating will be grounded in the culture of the person consulting the psychiatrist, the culture of their family or families, and the culture of the community in which they live and have their being. Yet culture itself is not static (see Chapter 1) and so the approach to mental health cannot be something that is fixed. In my view a system of psychiatry that is multicultural may use some form of diagnosis – or it may not – but the basic difference from the current unicultural psychiatry would be its flexibility. The narrow medical model would no longer dominate although it may play some part from time to time depending on circumstances. When mental health problems are evaluated, a total picture of the person and their family would be encompassed in the evaluation; categorisation of sorts may be used but not in terms of characteristics seen as unchangeable or fixed. In making an assessment, the psychiatrist would be led by whatever is important to the person who is the 'patient'. Thus, for many people the structures they are involved in (such as the social services system, housing market, etc.) may well be important, and for black and Asian people this includes racism in society. And racism in the consulting room and within the institution (i.e. psychiatric system itself) must not be ignored.

A psychiatry of the future that is multicultural clearly cannot be all things to every one but one thing that it must have are safeguards against racism that are effective *in practice*. Policies to counteract racism and encourage multicultural practice will be monitored by those affected – the users of services. The multiculturality of the discipline would be indicated by its openness to cultural diversity. Its anti-racism would be indicated by sensitivity of its practitioners to the actual experience of racism of service users, to the practitioners' prejudices, and to institutional racism in society.

I do not envisage a change in the basic approach of assessment (including a diagnosis), planning of therapy (hopefully in a treatment plan devised by a team in conjunction with the service users) and estimation of outcome (primarily by the service user and their families). Yet I see the value of diagnosis being superseded in importance by an understanding of the individual in the context of family and society. When a multicultural psychiatrist addresses the issues of 'therapy', a diversity of approaches will be considered in a context where an array of 'technologies' from all over the world with roots in many cultural traditions will be available (see Fernando 2002: 163–88). The use of western medication may still be the field that the psychiatrist has most knowledge about, but all other approaches will have credence and will be available within the multidisciplinary team providing care and therapy. The use of medication will be pragmatic (as described in Chapter 5) and worked out in conjunction with the service user. Outcome must finally be what the service user thinks it is. But clearly their viewpoints may have to be complemented by those of professionals running the services that they have accessed.

The training of psychiatrists and psychologists of the future – and of course the training of other disciplines in the mental health field – will have to be culturally broad based. They would need to include some basic knowledge of Asian, African and other psychologies, an understanding of a variety of illness concepts and ideologies regarding mental health, and a training in clinical methods that allows them to practise in such a way that the therapy is appropriate and meaningful for individuals and families from diverse backgrounds. Promoting multiculturalism and the struggle against racism are inextricably linked, and this will always be so. So the training in culture must be accompanied by a deep understanding of racism – personal racism and institutional racism – from both historical and experiential viewpoints. But more importantly, all practitioners must have an understanding of their own limitations, especially when they are dealing with people whose backgrounds are very different to their own, and an acknowledgement that psychiatry can never be precise and objective. The result of education and training based on such principles should result in psychiatrists who look primarily to the people they hope to help, their 'patients', for guidance and collaboration in working out the best approach to the (mental health) problems jointly identified in the course of an assessment.

My brief description of a multicultural psychiatry may seem vague and imprecise. But the lack of precision and extreme variability is its very essence. People's lives are not precisely defined and an assessment needs to address this very fact. As people's backgrounds and experiences vary, psychiatric approaches too must vary. And they must address problems as seen from the viewpoints of people who use the services in the light of *their* hope and fears. Clearly, a language will have to be developed to describe the multicultural assessments of a multicultural psychiatry but in this language diagnosis as currently envisaged must play a very minor part in a total assessment.

Flexible psychotherapy and counselling

Psychotherapy and counselling are, by and large, ethnocentric disciplines geared to ways of thinking and working that are almost exclusively (culturally) European. If psychotherapists and counsellors are to fulfil a useful role in the society for all who need their services, they must take on board the realities of working and living in a multicultural society. In other words, every effort must be made to bring into the theoretical frameworks that inform psychotherapy and counselling 'psychologies' from non-western sources, and to widen the approaches in professional practices so that they are sensitive to – in tune with – ways of thinking, behaving and relating that connect with the diversity of their clients and potential clients. And ways of working must address institutional racism.

Psychotherapy and counselling are closely tied up with western psychology. According to Pederson (1998) there have been three historical movements (or forces) within modern western psychology: The first was psychoanalytic theory that emphasized the power of unconscious forces, biological impulses and other processes within the individual; the second began when positivism and objectivity was emphasised leading to behaviourism; the third force was existentialism in Europe and humanism in the US promoting a positive view of human nature. Pederson goes on to suggest that multiculturalism is a 'fourth force' or dimension of western psychology 'that goes beyond the psychodynamic, behavioral, and humanistic perspectives' (1998: 3), to introduce a 'relativistic perspective' to all aspects of western psychology. I believe that Pederson underestimates the resistance to this force taking hold but, if he is right and this force does have an impact, it is difficult to determine how and to what extent it would affect the practical fields of psychotherapy and counselling. In my view, this force is not being felt very much in the British scene.

In Chapter 5, I propose some ways in which the training of psychotherapists and counsellors may change and I indicate changes in the way psychotherapy and counselling are practised. This is a start. If indeed, as Pederson suggests (see above), the fourth force of cultural relativity becomes embedded in psychology and then percolates through into psychotherapy and counselling, the scene in these disciplines may be much changed in the future. The danger is that such a force may not address some of the serious issues within psychotherapy and counselling that affect their use, if all it does is to bring about a (culturally) relativistic approach. In my view, in the present context of racism in society, there must be a revision of practices in psychotherapy and counselling so that the practitioners will actively incorporate an anti-racist dimension to their work, base their interpretations on an acknowledgement of a variety of psychologies, and be in a position to develop rapport with their clients by appreciating matters such as spirituality and connectedness in thinking (see pp. 115–17 and 125–7).

Meaningful psychiatric research

The fact that psychiatric research on 'ethnic issues' has, on the whole, been of very limited use if any at all (see Chapter 1) should carry lessons for the future. In Chapter 5 I suggest changes in both psychiatric research methods and the research agenda in mental health. Eventually, I hope to see psychiatric research being both useful in promoting changes that benefit users of psychiatric services and productive in furthering knowledge about the human condition from all dimensions: biological, social, psychological and spiritual. In the future, psychiatric research must be carefully vetted before being funded. Pharmaceutical companies should not be funding research directly but should be compelled to contribute resources to a national funding agency, largely controlled by a mixture of professionals and service users. The stage should be set then for pursuing research into techniques for alleviating distress whether these are based on neuropsychological, social or psychological approaches. In such research service users – people who have experienced the problems identified for research – should be closely involved in planning the research and guiding researchers because they are really in the best position to judge the sort of questions that research needs to find answers for. The primary focus for psychiatric research would be 'therapy' – at least for the purposes of the research protocol. Thus research would be exploring the use of a wide range of techniques such as drugs, exercise, yoga, talking therapies, etc., for alleviating what people themselves identify as problems (usually causing distress).

Research into mental health services in the future should be bottom-up rather than top-down; deficiencies and problems identified by users of services should form the basis for funded research into improving services, with professionals and other specialists contributing to the development of methods and strategies for research. Identifying the nature and extent of need will be based primarily on how these are seen by ordinary people from all communities. Some sort of categorisation may be required but the categories will be built up on the basis of problems and needs identified by communities. Epidemiology based on identifying 'illness' would, by then, have disappeared.

Summary

This final chapter envisages a multicultural psychiatry working within multicultural mental health services. Psychiatry and mental health services do not function in a social vacuum and so these disciplines will always need to address the nature of tensions in society and the institutionally racist nature of many of its systems. In a society that is culturally diverse, some of the tensions within it are likely to centre on differences between people seen in cultural and/or racial terms. In addressing institutional racism, mental health services cannot afford to ignore racism within its own structures and within the systems of psychiatry and psychology. In other words, psychiatry will always need to address the cultural diversity of society and racism in all its forms. In this chapter I look to a future when psychiatry and the mental health services take these issues on board fully, or almost fully, so that they provide appropriate services for everyone on an equitable, or nearly equitable, basis. The picture I present is of a psychiatric system that ensures that practitioners in the mental health field see people as people and not as carriers of 'illness' or 'health', taking account of their cultural backgrounds, working closely with users of services and actively counteracting racism. I believe that the future that I envisage is achievable.

References

Adams, F. (1856) (ed. and trans.) *The Extant Works of Aretaeus, the Cappadocian*. London: Sydenham Society.

Adams, W. and Kendell, R. E. (1996) 'Influenza and schizophrenia'. *British Journal of Psychiatry* 169: 252–3.

Adebimpe, V. R. (1994) 'Race, racism, and epidemiological surveys'. *Hospital and Community Psychiatry* 45(1): 27–31.

Agnivesa (1983) *Caraka Samhita* vol 1, 2nd edn, (trans. R. K. Sharma and V. B. Dash). Varanasi, India: Choukhamba Sanskrit Series Office.

Ahmad, W. I. U. (1989) 'Policies, pills and political will: critique of policies to improve the health status of ethnic minorities'. *Lancet* 1: 148–50.

—— (1993) 'Making black people sick: 'race', ideology and health research', in W. I. U. Ahmad (ed.) *'Race' and Health in Contemporary Britain*. Buckingham: Open University Press, pp. 11–33.

Allon, R. (1971) 'Sex, race, socio-economic status, social mobility, and process-reactive ratings of schizhophrenia'. *Journal of Nervous and Mental Disease* 153: 343–50.

Amarasingham, L. R. (1980) 'Movement among traditional healers in Sri Lanka; a case study of a Sinhalese patient'. *Culture, Medicine and Psychiatry* 4: 71–92.

Anon (1851) 'Startling facts from the census'. *American Journal of Insanity* 8(2): 153–5.

Anwar, M. and Ali, A. (1987) *Overseas Doctors. Experience and Expectations*. London: Commission for Racial Equality.

Audit Commission (2000) *Another Country. Implementing Dispersal under the Immigration and Asylum Act 1999*. London: The Audit Commission.

Babcock, J. W. (1895) 'The colored insane'. *Alienist and Neurologist* 16: 423–47.

Bagley, C. (1971) 'Mental illness in immigrant minorities in London'. *Journal of Biosocial Science* 3: 449–59.

Ballantyne, A. (1988) 'Young blacks vulnerable to schizophrenia'. *The Guardian*, 31 October 1988, p. 6.

Barnes, D. M. (1987) 'Biological issues in schizophrenia'. *Science* 235: 430–3.

Barnes, M. and Berke, J. (1971) *Two Accounts of a Journey Through Madness*. London: MacGibbon and Kee.

Baron, A. (2001) *An Indian Affair. From Riches to Raj*. London: Channel Four Books, Macmillan.

Barzun, J. (1965) *Race: A Study of Superstition*. New York: Harper and Row, cited by Husband, 1982.

Bateson, G., Jackson, D., Haley, J. and Weakland, J. (1956) 'Toward a theory of schizophrenia'. *Behavioural Science* 1: 251–64.

BBC (2001) First part of a three part series *Race, Culture and Creed*, Broadcast on Radio 4, 26 December 2001, London: British Broadcasting Corporation.

Bebbington, P. E., Hurry, J. and Tennant, C. (1981) 'Psychiatric disorders in selected immigrant groups in Camberwell'. *Social Psychiatry* 16: 43–51.

Beliappa, J. (1991) *Illness or Distress? Alternative Models of Mental Health*. London: Confederation of Indian Organisations.

Bentall, R. P. (1990) 'The syndromes and symptoms of psychosis', in R. P. Bentall (ed.) *Reconstructing Schizophrenia*. London and New York: Routledge, pp. 23–60.

——, Jackson, H. F. and Pilgrim, D. (1988) 'Abandoning the concept of "schizophrenia": Some implications of validity arguments for psychological research into psychotic phenomena'. *British Journal of Clinical Psychology* 27: 303–24.

——, Kaney, S. and Dewey, M. E. (1991) 'Paranoia and social reasoning: an attribution theory analysis'. *British Journal of Clinical Psychology* 30: 13–23.

Berrington, A. (1996) 'Marriage patterns and inter-ethnic unions', in D. Coleman and J. Salt (eds) *Ethnicity in the 1991 Census. Vol. 1: Demographic Characteristics of the Ethnic Minority Populations*. London: HMSO.

Berrios, G. E. (1987) 'Historical aspects of psychoses: nineteenth century issues'. *British Medical Bulletin* 43(3): 484–98.

—— and Chen, E. Y. H. (1993) 'Recognising psychiatric symptoms: relevance of diagnostic practice'. *British Journal of Psychiatry* 163: 308–14.

Berthoud, R. and Beishon, S. (1997) 'People, families and households', in T. Modood, R. Berthoud, J. Lakey, P. Smith, V. Satnam and S. Beishon (eds) *Ethnic Minorities in Britain. Diversity and Disadvantage*. London: Policy Studies Institute, pp. 18–59.

bhabha, homi k. (1994) *The Location of Culture*. London: Routledge.

Bhugra, D. (1992) 'Psychiatry in ancient Indian texts: a review'. *History of Psychiatry* iii: 167–86.

——, Leff, J., Mallett, R., Der, G., Corridan, B. and Rudge, S. (1997) 'Incidence and outcome of schizophrenia in Whites, African-Caribbeans and Asians in London'. *Psychological Medicine* 27: 791–8.

Bhui, K. (2002) 'London's ethnic minorities and the provision of mental health services', in K. Bhui (ed.) *Racism and Mental Health. Prejudice and Suffering.* London: Jessica Kingsley, pp. 139–87.

Bjorgo, T. (1997) '"The invaders", "the traitors" and "the resistance movement": the extreme right's conceptualisation of opponents and self in Scandinavia', in T. Modood and P. Werbner (eds) *The Politics of Multiculturalism in the New Europe: Racism, Identity and Community.* London: Zed Books, pp. 54–72.

Blackstock, C. (2002) 'Blunkett in clash over marriages'. *The Guardian*, 8 February 2002, p. 1.

Bleuler, E. (1911) *Dementia Præcox or the Group of Schizophrenias* (trans. J. Zitkin). New York: International Universities Press, reprinted 1950.

Bloch, S. and Reddaway, P. (1984) *The Shadows over World Psychiatry.* London: Gollancz.

Boedjarath, I. and van Bekkum, D. (1997) *Een blik in de transculturele hulpverlening. Vijftien jaar ervaring met verlies en verrijking.* Utrecht: Uitgeverij Jan van Arkel.

Bourne, J. (2001) 'The life and times of institutional racism'. *Race and Class* 43: 7–22.

Boyle, M. (2002) *Schizophrenia. A Scientific Delusion?* 2nd edn. London: Routledge.

Breggin, P. R. and Breggin, G. R. (1993) 'A biomedical programme for urban violence control in the US: the dangers of psychiatric social control'. *Changes* 11(1): 59–71.

Bright, T. (1586) *A Treatise of Melancholy.* London: Vautrolier.

Brightwell, R. (1989) Letter in *The Listener*, 13 April 1989, p. 18.

Bromberg, W. and Simon, F. (1968) 'The "protest" psychosis. A special type of reactive psychosis'. *Archives of General Psychiatry* 19: 155–60.

Brugha, T. S. (2002) 'Editorial: The end of the beginning: a requiem for the categorization of mental disorder?' *Psychological Medicine* 32: 1149–54.

Burnley Task Force (2001) *Burnley Independent Task Force Report* (chairman: Lord Anthony Clarke). Burnley, Lancashire: Burnley Borough Council.

Burton, R. (1621) *The Anatomy of Melancholy*, 11th edn. London: Hodson, 1806.

Bynum, W. F. Jr. (1981) 'Rationales for therapy in British psychiatry, 1780–1835', in A. Scull (ed.) *Madhouses, Mad-doctors and Madmen: The Social History of Psychiatry in the Victorian Era.* London: Athlone Press, pp. 35–57.

Campling, P. (1989) 'Race, culture and psychotherapy'. *Psychiatric Bulletin* 13: 550–1.

Cannon, M. (2001) 'Highlights of this issue'. *British Journal of Psychiatry* 178: 191.

Cannon, M., Cotter, D., Coffey, V. P., *et al.* (1996) 'Prenatal exposure to the 1957 influenza epidemic and adult schizophrenia: a follow-up study'. *British Journal of Psychiatry* 168: 368–71.

Capra, F. (1982) *The Turning Point. Science, Society, and the Rising Culture.* London: Wildwood House.

Carf (Campaign against Racism and Fascism) (1997) 'Commentary'. *Race and Class* 39(1): 85–95.

Carmichael, S. and Hamilton, C. V. (1967) *Black Power. The Politics of Liberation in America.* New York: Random House.

Carothers, J. C. (1953) *The African Mind in Health and Disease. A Study in Ethnopsychiatry.* WHO Monograph Series No. 17. Geneva: World Health Organisation.

Carpenter, L. and Brockington, I. F. (1980) 'A study of mental illness in Asians, West Indians and Africans living in Manchester'. *British Journal of Psychiatry* 137: 201–5.

Cartwright, S. A. (1851) 'Report on the diseases and physical peculiarities of the Negro race'. *New Orleans Medical and Surgical Journal* May 1851: 691–715. Reprinted in A. C. Caplan, H. T. Engelhardt and J. J. McCartney (eds) (1981) *Concepts of Health and Disease.* Massachusets: Addison-Wesley.

Cashmore, E. (1979) *Rastaman. The Rastafarian Movement in England.* London: Allen and Unwin.

Chaplin, R. (2000) 'Psychiatrists can cause stigma too'. Letter in *British Journal of Psychiatry* 177: 467.

Charlton, B. (2000) *Psychiatry and the Human Condition.* Abingdon, Oxon: Radcliffe Medical Press.

Cochrane, R. (1977) 'Mental illness in immigrants in England and Wales: an analysis of mental hospital admissions, 1971'. *Social Psychiatry* 12: 23–35.

Cohen, P. (1999) *New Ethnicities, Old Racisms?* London: Zed Books.

Coker, N. (ed.) (2001) *Racism in Medicine. An Agenda for Change.* London: King's Fund Publishing.

Collins, M. (2001) 'Racial harassment in the NHS', in N. Coker (ed.) *Racism in Medicine. An Agenda for Change.* London: King's Fund Publishing, pp. 169–90.

Commission for Racial Equality (1983) *Ethnic Minority Hospital Staff.* London: Commission for Racial Equality.

—— (1987) *Racial Attacks. A Survey in Eight Areas of Britain.* London: Commission for Racial Equality.

Conze, E. (1957) *Buddhism. Its Essence and Development* 3rd edn. Oxford: Bruno Cassirer.

Cooper, D. (1970) *Psychiatry and Anti-Psychiatry*. London: Paladin.

Cox, J. (2001) 'Commentary: institutional racism in British psychiatry'. *Psychiatric Bulletin* 25: 248–9.

Crass, S. (2000) *Real Shame*. www.peoplewho.org/readingroom/caras. stigma.htm

Crisp, A. H. (2000) 'Changing minds: every family in the land. An update on the College's campaign'. *Psychiatric Bulletin* 24: 267–8.

Crocker, I., Major, B. and Steele, C. (1998) 'Social stigma', in D. T. Gilbert, S. T. Fiske and G. Lindzey (eds) *The Handbook of Social Psychology, Vol. 2*, 4th edn. Boston, MA: McGraw-Hill, pp. 504–53.

Crow, T. J. and Done, D. J. (1992) 'Prenatal exposure to influenza does not cause schizophrenia'. *British Journal of Psychiatry* 161: 390–3.

Dalal, F. (1988) 'The racism of Jung'. *Race and Class* 29(3): 1–22.

Damasio, A. R. (1996) *Descartes' Error. Emotion, Reason and the Human Brain*. London: Macmillan.

D'Ardenne, P. and Mahtani, A. (1999) *Transcultural Counselling in Action* 2nd edn. London: Sage.

Dean, G., Walsh, D., Downing, H. and Shelley, E. (1981) 'First admissions of native-born and immigrants to psychiatric hospitals in South-East England, 1970'. *British Journal of Psychiatry* 139: 506–12.

Defendorf, A. (1902) *Clinical Psychiatry. A Textbook for Students and Physicians* (abstracted and adapted from the 6th German edn of Kraepelin's *Lehrbuch der Psychiatrie*). New York: Macmillan.

Delay, J., Deniker, P. and Harl, J. M. (1957) 'Utilisation en thérapeutique psychiatrique d'une phenothiazine d'action centrale élective (4560 RP). *Annals of Medical Psychology* (Paris) 110: 112–17.

Department of Health (1999) *National Service Framework for Mental Health. Modern Standards and Service Models*. London: Department of Health.

—— (2002) *Draft Mental Health Bill*. Cm 5528-1, London: The Stationery Office.

Department of Health and Home Office (1994) *Review of Health and Social Services for Mentally Disordered Offenders and Others Requiring Similar Services, Vol. 6, Race, Gender and Equal Opportunities*. London: HMSO (chairman, Dr John Reed).

Devereux, G. (1939) 'Mohave culture and personality'. *Character and Personality* 8: 91–109.

Dickenson, D. and Fulford, K. W. M. (2000) *In Two Minds. A Casebook of Psychiatric Ethics*. Oxford: Oxford University Press.

Dols, M. W. (1992) *Majnūn: The Madman in Medieval Islamic Society* D. E. Immisch (ed.). Oxford: Clarendon Press.

Donald, A. (2001) 'The Wal-Marting of American psychiatry: an ethnography of psychiatric practice in the late twentieth century'. *Culture, Medicine and Psychiatry* 25(4): 427–39.

Du Bois, W. E. B. (1970) *The Souls of Black Folk*. New York: Washington Square Press (first published by McClurg, Chicago 1903).

Eagles, J. M. (1991) 'The relationship between schizophrenia and immigration. Are there alternatives to psychosocial hypotheses?' *British Journal of Psychiatry* 159: 783–9.

Eagleton, T. (2000) *The Idea of Culture*. Oxford: Blackwell.

Eaton, W. W. and Harrison, G. (2000) 'Epidemiology, social deprivation, and community psychiatry'. *Current Opinion in Psychiatry* 13: 185–7.

Editorial (2001) 'Inside our changing land'. In 'Race in Britain', special edition of *The Observer*, 25 November 2001, p. 1.

Eleftheriadou, Z. (1994) *Transcultural Counselling*. London: Central Book Publishing.

Engel, G. K. (1977) 'The need for a new medical model: a challenge for biomedicine'. *Science* 196: 129–36.

Esmail, A. (2001) 'Racial discrimination in medical schools', in N. Coker (ed.) *Racism in Medicine. An Agenda for Change*. London: King's Fund, pp. 81–97.

Essed, P. (1990) *Everyday Racism* 2nd edn (trans. C. Jaffé). Alameda, CA: Hunter House. (Originally published in Dutch as *Alledaags Racisme*. Baarn, The Netherlands: Ambo.)

European Commission (1997) *Racism and Xenophobia*. Draft final report presented at the closing Conference of the European Year Against Racism, Luxembourg 18 and 19 December 1997. Strasbourg: European Commission.

European Union Institutions (2001) *Commission Proposes EU-wide Approximation of Penal Laws on Racist Offences*. Press release, 28 November 2001. http://europa.eu.int

Eze, E. C. (1997) 'Introduction', in E. C. Eze (ed.) *Race and the Enlightenment. A Reader*. Cambridge, MA and Oxford: Blackwell, pp. 1–9.

Fabrega, H. (1991a) 'The culture and history of psychiatric stigma in early modern and modern western societies: a review of recent literature'. *Comprehensive Psychiatry* 32(2): 97–119.

—— (1991b) 'Psychiatric stigma in non-western societies'. *Comprehensive Psychiatry* 32: 534–51.

Fanon, F. (1952) *Peau Noire, Masques Blancs*. Paris: Editions de Seuil (trans. C. L. Markmann *Black Skin, White Masks*. Grove Press, New York 1967).

—— (1967) 'Racism and culture' (text of Frantz Fanon's speech before the first congress of Negro writers and artists in Paris, September 1965, and published in the special issue of *Présence Africaine*, June–November, 1956), in F. Maspero (ed.) *Toward the African Revolution. Political Essays* (trans. H. Chevalier), New York: Grove Press, pp. 31–44.

Favazza, A. R. (1985) 'Anthropology and psychiatry', in H. I. Kaplan and B. J. Sadock (eds) *Comprehensive Textbook of Psychiatry*, 4th edn, vol. 1. Baltimore: Williams and Wilkins, pp. 247–65.

Fernando, S. (1988) *Race and Culture in Psychiatry*. London: Croom Helm (published as paperback by Routledge, 1989).

—— (1989) 'Personality clash', Letter in *The Listener* 30 March 1989, p. 19.

—— (1991) 'Racial stereotypes'. *British Journal of Psychiatry* 158: 289–90.

—— (ed.) (1995a) *Mental Health in a Multi-ethnic Society*. London: Routledge.

—— (1995b) 'Social realities and mental health', in S. Fernando (ed.) *Mental Health in a Multi-ethnic Society*. London: Routledge, pp. 11–35.

—— (1995c) 'Professional interventions; therapy and care', in S. Fernando (ed.) *Mental Health in a Multi-ethnic Society*. London: Routledge, pp. 36–49.

—— (1995d) 'The way forward', in S. Fernando (ed.) *Mental Health in a Multi-ethnic Society*. London: Routledge, pp. 193–216.

—— (1996) 'Black people working in white institutions: lessons from personal experience'. *Human Systems: The Journal of Systemic Consultation and Management* 7(2–3): 143–54.

—— (1998a) 'Open letter to Frank Dobson'. *Openmind* 94: November/ December, 15.

—— (1998b) 'Modern schizophrenia and racism', in S. Fernando, D. Ndegwa and M. Wilson (eds) *Forensic Psychiatry, Race and Culture*. London: Routledge, pp. 51–66.

—— (1998c) 'Anger, criminality and dangerousness', in S. Fernando, D. Ndegwa and M. Wilson (eds) *Forensic Psychiatry, Race and Culture*. London: Routledge, pp. 67–80.

—— (2002) *Mental Health, Race and Culture* 2nd edn. London: Palgrave.

——, Ndegwa, D. and Wilson, M. (eds) (1998) *Forensic Psychiatry, Race and Culture*. London: Routledge.

Ferns, P. and Dutt, R. (1999) *Letting Through Light*. London: The Race Equality Unit.

Ferns, P. and Madden, M. (1995) 'Training to promote equality', in S. Fernando (ed.) *Mental Health in a Multi-ethnic Society*. London: Routledge, pp. 107–19.

Field, M. J. (1958) 'Mental disorder in rural Ghana'. *Journal of Mental Science* 104: 1043–51.

Fitzpatrick, P. (1990) 'Racism and the innocence of law', in D. T. Goldberg (ed.) *Anatomy of Racism*. Minneapolis, MN: University of Minnesota Press, pp. 247–62.

Flaskerud, J. H. and Hu, L. (1992) 'Relationship between ethnicity and psychiatric diagnosis'. *The Journal of Nervous and Mental Disease* 180: 296–303.

Foucault, M. (1967) *Madness and Civilisation* (trans. R. Howard). London: Tavistock (first published in French as *Historie de la Folie*, 1961, by Librairie Plon).

—— (1988) *Politics Philosophy Culture. Interviews and Other Writings 1977–1984* L. D. Kritzman (ed.). London: Routledge.

Frable, D. E. S. (1993) 'Dimensions of marginality: distinctions among those who are different'. *Personal and Social Psychology Bulletin* 19(4): 370–80.

Frank, J. D. (1963) *Persuasion and Healing*. New York: Schoken Books.

Franklin, A. J. (2002) 'Raising boys into men: challenges to families of black male youth'. Talk given on 26 April at the *Visibility and Invisibility* conference held at Leeds, UK.

Frawley, D. (1989) *Ayurvedic Healing: A Comprehensive Guide*. Delhi: Motilal Banarsidass Publishers.

Freud, S. (1913) *Totem and Taboo. Some Points of Agreement between Mental Lives of Savages and Neurotics*. Vienna: Hugo Heller (trans. and published in English by Routledge and Kegan Paul, London, 1950).

Freud, S. (1917) 'Mourning and melancholia', in J. Strachey (ed.) *The Standard Edition of the Complete Psychological Works of Sigmund Freud Vol. 14* (trans. from the German under the General Editorship of J. Strachey in collaboration with A. Freud assisted by A. Strachey and A. Tyson). London: Hogarth Press, 1957, pp. 243–58.

Friedman, S. and Paradis, C. (2002) 'Panic disorder in African-Americans: symptomatology and isolated sleep paralysis'. *Culture, Medicine and Psychiatry* 26: 179–98.

Fromm, E. (1976) *To have or to be?* London: Jonathan Cape.

——, Suzuki, D. T. and de Martino, R. (1960) *Zen Buddhism and Psychoanalysis*. London: George Allen and Unwin.

Fryer, P. (1984) *Staying Power. The History of Black People in Britain*. London: Pluto Press.

Fulford, K. W. M., Smirnov, A. Y. U. and Snow, E. (1993) 'Concepts of disease and the abuse of psychiatry in the USSR'. *British Journal of Psychiatry* 162: 801–10.

Gergen, K. J. (1973) 'Social psychology as history'. *Journal of Personality and Social Psychology* 26: 309–20.

Gill, P. S. (2001) 'General practitioners, ethnic diversity and racism', in N. Coker (ed.) *Racism in Medicine. An Agenda for Change*. London: King's Fund, pp. 99–120.

Gillis, L. S. (1977) Letter to the editor. *Lancet* 2: 920–1.

Goel, K. M., Campbell, S., Logan, R. W., Sweet, E. M., Attenburrow, A. and Arneil, G. C. (1981) 'Reduced prevalence of rickets in Asian children in Glasgow'. *Lancet* 2: 405–7.

Goffman, E. (1968) *Stigma. Notes on the Management of Spoiled Identity*. Harmondsworth: Penguin Books.

Goldberg, D. T. (1993) *Racist Culture. Philosophy and the Politics of Meaning.* Oxford: Blackwell.

Goldberg, D. T. and Essed, P. (2002) 'Introduction', in *Race Critical Theories.* Malden, MA and Oxford: Blackwell, pp. 1–11.

Gordon, P. (1986) *Racial Violence and Harassment.* London: Runnymede Trust.

—— (1989) *Fortress Europe? The Meaning of 1992.* London: Runnymede Trust.

Gorman, G. (1995) 'Qalb'. *Openmind,* 76: 19.

Gottesman, I. I. (1991) *Schizophrenia Genesis. The Origins of Madness.* New York: Freeman.

Green, E. M. (1914) 'Psychoses among Negroes – a comparative study'. *Journal of Nervous and Mental Disorder* 41: 697–708.

Grier, W. H. and Cobbs, P. M. (1969) *Black Rage.* New York: Bantam Books (first published by Basic Books, London 1968).

Grob, G. N. (1983) *Mental Illness and American Society 1875–1940.* Princeton, NJ: Princeton University Press.

Haasen, C., Lambert, M. and Yagdiran, O. (1996) 'Diagnostic aspects of psychiatric disorders among migrants'. *Curare* 19(2): 347–52.

Haghighat, R. (2001) 'A unitary theory of stigmatisation'. *British Journal of Psychiatry* 178: 207–15.

Haley, J. (1963) *Strategies of Psychotherapy.* New York: Grune and Stratton.

Hall, G. S. (1904) *Adolescence its Psychology and its Relations to Physiology, Anthropology, Sociology, Sex, Crime, Religion and Education* vol. II. New York: D. Appleton.

Hall, S. (1980) 'Race, articulation and societies structured in dominance', in UNESCO (ed.) *Sociological Theories: Race and Colonialism.* Paris: UNESCO, pp. 305–45 (reprinted in Goldberg, D. T. and Essed, P. (eds) (2002) *Race Critical Theories,* Malden MA and Oxford: Blackwell, pp. 38–68).

—— (1992) 'New ethnicities', in J. Donald and A. Rattansi (eds) *'Race', Culture and Difference.* London: Sage, pp. 252–9.

——, Critcher, C., Jefferson, T., Clarke, J. and Roberts, B. (1978) *Policing the Crisis. Mugging, The State, and Law and Order.* London: Macmillan.

Hammer, L. (1990) *Dragon Rises, Red Bird Flies. Psychology and Chinese Medicine.* New York: Station Hill Press.

Harari, E. (2001) 'Whose evidence? Lessons from the philosophy of science and the epistemology of medicine'. *Australian and New Zealand Journal of Psychiatry* 35: 724–30.

Harding, C. (ed.) (1995) *Not just Black and White.* An information pack about mental health services for people from Black communities, London: Good Practices in Mental Health.

Hare, E. (1988) 'Schizophrenia as a recent disease'. *British Journal of Psychiatry* 153: 521–31.

Harrison, G. (1990) 'Searching for the causes of schizophrenia; the role of migrant studies'. *Schizophrenia Bulletin* 16: 663–71.

——, Glazebrook, C., Brewin, J., Cantwell, R., *et al.* (1997) 'Increased incidence of psychotic disorders in migrants from the Caribbean to the United Kingdom'. *Psychological Medicine* 27: 799–806.

——, Ineichen, B., Smith, J. and Morgan, H. G. (1984) 'Psychiatric hospital admissions in Bristol. II. Social and clinical aspects of compulsory admission'. *British Journal of Psychiatry* 145: 605–11.

——, Owens, D., Holton, A., Neilson, D. and Boot, D. (1988) 'A prospective study of severe mental disorder in Afro-Caribbean patients'. *Psychological Medicine* 18: 643–57.

Hays, P. (1984) 'The nosological status of schizophrenia'. *Lancet* 1: 1342–5.

Healy, D. (1990a) *The Suspended Revolution. Psychiatry and Psychotherapy Re-examined.* London and Boston: Faber and Faber.

—— (1990b) 'The new science of insanity'. *New Scientist* 6 October 1990, pp. 34–7.

Hegemann, T. and Salman, R. (2001) *Transkulturelle Psychiatrie. Konzepte für die Arbeit mit Menschen aus anderen Kulturen.* Bonn: Psychiatrie Verlag.

Hes, J. P. (1960) 'Manic-depressive illness in Israel'. *American Journal of Psychiatry* 116: 1082–6.

Home Department (1999) *The Stephen Lawrence Inquiry. Report of an Inquiry by Sir William Macpherson of Cluny.* CM4262-I, London: The Stationery Office.

Home Office (1976) *Racial Discrimination. A Guide to the Race Relations Act 1976.* London: Home Office.

—— (1981) *The Brixton Disorders 10–12 April 1981. Report of an Inquiry by the Rt. Hon. The Lord Scarman.* Cmnd 8427, London: Her Majesty's Stationery Office.

—— (1998) *Fairer, Faster and Firmer: A Modern Approach to Immigration and Asylum.* London: The Stationery Office.

—— (2000) *Race Equality in Public Services.* London: Home Office.

—— (2001) *Race Relations (Amendment) Act 2000. New Laws for Successful Multi-Racial Britain. Proposals for Implementation.* London: Home Office.

—— (2002a) *Race and the Criminal Justice System.* A publication under Section 95 of the Criminal Justice Act 1991, London: Home Office.

—— (2002b) *Secure Borders, Safe Haven. Integration with Diversity in Modern Britain.* CM 5387, London: The Stationery Office.

hooks, bell (1994) *Outlaw Culture. Resisting Representations.* New York: Routledge.

Howitt, D. and Owusu-Bempah, J. (eds) (1994) *The Racism of Psychology. Time for Change*. London: Harvester Wheatsheaf.

Hunter, R. A. and MacAlpine, I. (1963) *Three Hundred Years of Psychiatry 1535–1860: A History Presented in Selected English Texts*. London: Oxford University Press.

Husband, C. (1982) '"Race", the continuity of a concept', in C. Husband (ed.) *Race in Britain. Continuity and Change*. London: Hutchinson, pp. 11–23.

Huxley, A (1947) 'Introduction', in S. Prabhavandanda and C. Isherwood (eds and trans) *The Song of God. Bhagavad-Gita*. London: Phoenix House, pp. 5–19.

Independent Review Team (2001) *Community Cohesion: A Report of the Independent Review Team Chaired by Ted Cantle*. London: Home Office.

Ineichen, B., Harrison, G. and Morgan, H. G. (1984) 'Psychiatric hospital admissions in Bristol. 1. Geographical and ethnic factors'. *British Journal of Psychiatry* 145: 600–4.

Ingleby, D. (1980) 'Understanding mental illness', in D. Ingleby (ed.) *Critical Psychiatry. The Politics of Mental Health*. New York: Pantheon Books, pp. 23–71.

Institute of Race Relations (1991) *Deadly Silence. Black Deaths in Custody*. London: Institute of Race Relations.

—— (2002a) 'France'. *European Race Bulletin* 39: 6–9.

—— (2002b) 'Germany'. *European Race Bulletin* 39: 9–15.

Ito, K. L. and Maranba, G. G. (2002) 'Therapeutic beliefs of Asian American therapists: views from an ethnic-specific clinic'. *Transcultural Psychiatry* 39(1): 33–73.

Jackson, S. W. (1986) *Melancholia and Depression. From Hippocratic Times to Modern Times*. New Haven and London: Yale University Press.

Jaco, E. G. (1960) *Social Epidemiology of Mental Disorders. A Psychiatric Survey of Texas*. New York: Russell Sage Foundation.

Jadhav, S. (2000) 'The cultural construction of western depression', in V. Skultans and J. Cox (eds) *Anthropological Approaches to Psychological Medicine. Crossing Bridges*. London: Jessica Kingsley, pp. 41–65.

Jadhav, S. and Littlewood, R. (1994) 'Defeat depression campaign: some medical anthropological queries'. *Psychiatric Bulletin* 18: 572–3.

Jaggi, O. P. (1981) *Ayurveda: Indian System of Medicine* 2nd edn, vol. 4. Delhi: Atma Ram and Sons.

Jarvis, E. (1853) 'On the supposed increase of insanity'. *American Journal of Insanity* 8: 333–64.

Jenner, F. A., Monteiro, A. C. D., Zagalo-Cardoso, J. A. and Cunha-Oliveira, J. A. (1993) *Schizophrenia. A Disease or Some Ways of Being Human?* Sheffield: Sheffield Academic Press.

Jennings, S. (1996) 'Developing black mental provision: challenging inequalities in partnership'. *Journal of Community and Applied Social Psychology* 6: 335–40.

Johnstone, E. C. (1999) 'Preface', in E. C. Johnstone, M. S. Humpreys, F. H. Lang, S. M. Lawrie and R. Sandler (eds) *Schizophrenia. Concepts and Clinical Management.* Cambridge: Cambridge University Press, pp. ix–xiv.

Jones, E. E., Farina, A., Hastorf, A. H., Markus, H., Miller, D. T. and Scott, R. A. (1984) *Social Stigma: The Psychology of Marked Relationships.* New York: Freeman, cited by Kurzban and Leary (2001).

Jones, M. (1968) *Social Psychiatry in Practice.* Harmondsworth: Penguin.

Jones, W. H. S. (1823) *Hippocrates with an English Translation.* London: Heinemann.

Jung. C. G. (1930) 'Your Negroid and Indian behaviour'. *Forum* 83(4): 193–9.

Jung, C. G. (1939) 'The dreamlike world of India'. *Asia (New York)* 39(1): 5–8 (reprinted in H. Read, M. Fordham and G. Adler (eds) *Civilization in Transition. Collected Works of C. G. Jung* vol. 10, London: Routledge and Kegan Paul (1964), 515–24).

Kakar, S. (1984) *Shamans, Mystics and Doctors. A Psychological Inquiry into India and its Healing Tradition.* London: Unwin Paperbacks.

—— (1995) 'Modern psychotherapies in traditional cultures: India, China, and Japan', in S. Kang (ed.) *Psychotherapy East and West. Integration of Psychotherapies.* Seoul: Korean Academy of Psychotherapy, pp. 79–85.

Kaptchuk, T. J. (1983) *Chinese Medicine.* London: Century Paperbacks.

Kareem, J. and Littlewood, R. (2000) *Intercultural Therapy* 2nd edn. Oxford: Blackwell Science.

Kendell, R. E. (1975) *The Role of Diagnosis in Psychiatry.* Oxford: Blackwell.

—— (1989) 'Clinical validity'. *Psychological Medicine* 19: 45–55.

—— and Kemp, I. W. (1989) 'Maternal influenza in the aetiology of schizophrenia'. *Archives of General Psychiatry* 46: 878–82.

King, D. J. and Cooper, S. J. (1989) 'Viruses, immunity and mental disorder'. *British Journal of Psychiatry* 154: 1–7.

King, M., Coker, E., Leavey, G., Hoar, A. and Johnson-Sabine, E. (1994) 'Incidence of psychotic illness in London: comparison of ethnic groups'. *British Medical Journal* 309: 1115–19.

Kleinman, A. (1977) 'Depression, somatization and the "new cross-cultural psychiatry"'. *Social Science and Medicine* 11: 3–10.

—— and Good, B. (eds) (1985) *Culture and Depression. Studies in the Anthropology and Cross-Cultural Psychiatry of Affect and Disorder.* Berkeley: University of California Press.

Koffman, J., Fulop, N. J., Pashley, D. and Coleman, K. (1997) 'Ethnicity and use of acute psychiatric beds: one-day survey in North and South Thames Regions'. *British Journal of Psychiatry* 171: 238–41.

Kraepelin, E. (1896) *Psychiatrie* 5th edn. Leipzig: Barth.

—— (1904) 'Vergleichende psychiatrie'. *Zentralblatt Nervenheilkunde und Psychiatrie* 27: 433–7 (trans. H. Marshall, in S. R. Hirsch and M. Shepherd (eds) *Themes and Variations in European Psychiatry*. Bristol: John Wright (1974), pp. 3–6).

—— (1919) 'Dementia præcox and paraphrenia' (trans. R. M. Barclay) in G. M. Robertson (ed.) *Textbook of Psychiatry* 8th edn. Edinburgh: Livingstone.

—— (1921) 'Manic depressive insanity and paranoia' (trans. R. M. Barclay) in G. M. Robertson (ed.) *Textbook of Psychiatry* 8th edn. Edinburgh: Livingstone.

Kraus, R. F. (1968) 'Cross-cultural validation of psychoanalytic theories of depression'. *Pennsylvania Psychiatric Quarterly* 3(8): 24–33 (cited by Obeyesekere, 1985).

Krishna, B. M. (2002) 'South Asians main targets of Sept. 11'. *South Asian-American Focus. India-West Newspaper* 15 March 2002, p. 1. http://www.ncomline.com/content/ncm/2002/mar/0315southasian.html

Kuller, L. H. (1999) 'Invited commentary: circular epidemiology'. *American Journal of Epidemiology* 150(9): 897–903.

Kurzban, R. and Leary, M. R. (2001) 'Evolutionary origins of stigmatization: the functions of social exclusion'. *Psychological Bulletin* 127(2): 187–208.

Lago, C. and Thompson, J. (1996) *Race, Culture and Counselling*. Buckingham: Open University Press.

Lambo, A. (1969) 'Traditional African cultures and Western medicine', in F. N. L. Poynter (ed.) *Medicine and Culture*. London: Wellcome Institute of the History of Medicine, pp. 201–10.

Larsson, S. (1991) 'Swedish racism: the democratic way'. *Race and Class* 32(3): 102–11.

Lau, A. and Zane, N. (2000) 'Examining the effects of ethnic-specific services: an analysis of cost-utilization and treatment outcomes for Asian American clients'. *Journal of Community Psychology* 28: 63–77.

Lawson, W. B., Hepler, N., Hollady, J. and Cuffal, B. (1994) 'Ethnicity as a factor in inpatient and outpatient admissions and diagnosis'. *Hospital and Community Psychiatry* 45: 72–4.

Leading Article (1977) 'Apartheid and mental health care'. *Lancet* 2: 491.

Lebra, W. P. (ed.) (1976) *Culture-bound Syndromes, Ethnopsychiatry and Alternate Therapies*. Honolulu: University of Hawaii Press.

Leff, J. (1973) 'Culture and the differentiation of emotional states'. *British Journal of Psychiatry* 123: 299–306.

—— (1981) *Psychiatry around the Globe. A Transcultural View*. New York: Marcel Dekker.

Leighton, A. H. and Hughes, J. M. (1961) 'Cultures as causative of mental disorder'. *Millbank Memorial Fund Quarterly* 39(3): 446–70.

Levy-Bruhl, L. (1923) *Primitive Mentality* (trans. L. A. Clare). London: Allen and Unwin.

Lewis, A. (1965) 'Chairman's opening remarks', in A. V. S. De Rueck and R. Porter (eds) *Transcultural Psychiatry. A Ciba Foundation Symposium.* London: Churchill, pp. 1–3.

Lewis, G., Croft-Jeffreys, C. and David, A. (1990) 'Are British psychiatrists racist?' *British Journal of Psychiatry* 157: 410–15.

Lieberman, J. A. and Koreen, A. R. (1993) 'Neurochemistry and neuroendocrinology of schizophrenia: a selective review'. *Schizophrenia Bulletin* 19: 371–429.

Linburg-Okken, A. (1989) *Migranten in de Psychiatrie.* Deventer, The Netherlands: Van Loghum Slaterus.

Lindsey, K. P. and Paul, G. L. (1989) 'Involuntary commitments to public mental institutions: issues involving the overrepresentation of Blacks and assessment of relevant functioning'. *Psychological Bulletin* 106(2): 171–83.

Littlewood, R. (1988) 'Cultural variation in the stigmatisation of mental illness'. *Lancet* 352: 1056–7.

—— (1989) 'Towards an intercultural therapy', in J. Kareem and R. Littlewood (eds) *Intercultural Therapy. Themes Interpretations and Practice.* London: Blackwell Science, pp. 3–13.

—— and Lipsedge, M. (1982) *Aliens and Alienists. Ethnic Minorities and Psychiatry.* Harmondsworth: Penguin.

Logan, M. H. (1979) 'Variations regarding Susto causality among the Cakchiquel of Guatemala'. *Culture, Medicine and Psychiatry* 3: 153–66.

Lombroso, C. (1911) *Crime: Its Causes and Remedies* (trans. H. P. Horton). London: Heinemann.

López Piñero, J. M. (1983) *Historical Origins of the Concept of Neurosis* (trans. D. Berrios). Cambridge: Cambridge University Press.

Loring, M. and Powell, B. (1988) 'Gender, race and DSM-III: a study of the objectivity of psychiatric diagnostic behavior'. *Journal of Health and Social Behavior* 29: 1–22.

Lucas, J. (1994) 'Race and Culture in Europe'. *Openmind* 69: June/July, 18.

Lyon, H. M., Kaney, S. and Bentall, R. P. (1994) 'The defensive function of persecutory delusions. Evidence from attribution tasks'. *British Journal of Psychiatry* 164: 637–46.

Lyons, B. G. (1971) *Voices of Melancholy.* London: Routledge and Kegan Paul.

Major, L. E. (2002) 'Incredible islands. A disturbing report shows universities must tackle race issues'. *Guardian Education*, 15 January 2002, p. 9.

Malik, Kenan (1996) *The Meaning of Race. Race, History and Culture in Western Society.* Basingstoke: Macmillan.

Malzberg, B. (1931) 'Mental disease among Jews. A second study'. *Mental Hygiene (New York)* 15: 766–74.

Malzberg, B. (1962) 'The distribution of mental disease according to religious affiliation in New York State 1940–1951'. *Mental Hygiene (New York)* 46: 510–22.

Marsella, A. J. (1978) 'Thought on cross-cultural studies on the epidemiology of depression'. *Culture, Medicine and Psychiatry* 2: 343–57.

—— (1980) 'Depression experience and disorder across cultures', in H. Triandis and J. Draguns (eds) *Handbook of Cross-Cultural Psychology* vol. 6. Rockleigh, NJ: Allyn and Bacon, pp. 237–89.

—— (1982) 'Culture and mental health: an overview', in A. J. Marsella and G. M. White (eds) *Cultural Conceptions of Mental Health and Therapy*. Dordrecht, Holland: Reidel, pp. 359–88.

Marshall, R. (1995) 'Schizophrenia. A constructive analogy or a convenient construct?', in J. Ellwood (ed.) *Psychosis. Understanding and Treatment*. London: Jessica Kingsley, pp. 54–69.

Maudsley, H. (1867) *The Physiology and Pathology of Mind*. New York: D. Appleton.

—— (1879) *The Pathology of Mind*. London: Macmillan.

May, J. V. (1922) *Mental Disease. A Public Health Problem*. Boston: Gorham.

McBride, E. (1988) 'Western civilisation: from Plato to Nato'. *The Activist* 21: 7 (cited by Pieterse, 1991).

McCauley, M. (2002) 'Home treatment service'. *Psychiatric Bulletin* 26: 155.

McCulloch, J. (1983) *Black Soul White Artifact. Fanon's Clinical Psychology and Social Theory*. Cambridge: Cambridge University Press.

McGorry, P. D. (1991) 'Paradigm failure in functional psychosis: review and implications'. *Australian and New Zealand Journal of Psychiatry* 25: 43–55.

McGovern, D. and Cope, R. (1987) 'The compulsory detention of males of different ethnic groups, with special reference to offender patients'. *British Journal of Psychiatry* 150: 505–12.

McManus, I. C. (1998) 'Factors affecting the likelihood of applicants being offered a place in medical schools in the United Kingdom in 1996 and 1997: retrospective study'. *British Medical Journal* 317: 1111–16.

Mednick, S. A., Machon, R. A., Huttanen, M. O. and Bonett, D. (1989) 'Adult schizophrenia following prenatal exposure to an influenza epidemic'. *Archives of General Psychiatry* 45: 189–92.

Mehta, D. K. (2002) *British National Formulary*. London: British Medical Association and Royal Pharmaceutical Society of Great Britain.

Mehta, G. (1980) *Karma Cola. The Marketing of the Mystic East*. London: Jonathan Cape.

Meldrum, A. (2001) 'Masakadza is great hope of change'. *The Guardian*, 25 September, p. 26.

Melotti, U. (1997) 'International migration in Europe; social projects and political cultures', in T. Modood and P. Werbner (eds) *The Politics of Multiculturalism in the New Europe: Racism, Identity and Community*. London: Zed Books, pp. 73–92.

Mental Health Act Commission (1987) *Second Biennial Report 1985–87*. London: HMSO.

—— (1989) *Third Biennial Report 1987–1989*. London: HMSO.

—— (1991) *Fourth Biennial Report 1989–1991*. London: HMSO.

—— (1993) *Fifth Biennial Report 1991–1993*. London: HMSO.

—— (1995) *Sixth Biennial Report 1993–1995*. London: HMSO.

—— (1997) *Seventh Biennial Report 1995–1997*. London: HMSO.

Meyer, A. (1905) 'Society Proceedings. New York Neurological Society'. *Journal of Nervous and Mental Disease* 32: 112–20.

Minuchin, S. and Fishman, H. C. (1981) *Family Therapy Techniques*. Cambridge, MA: Harvard University Press.

Modood, T. (1997) 'Employment', in T. Modood, R. Berthoud, J. Lakey, P. Smith, V. Satnam and S. Beishon (eds) *Ethnic Minorities in Britain. Diversity and Disadvantage*. London: Policy Studies Institute, pp. 83–149.

Monbiot, G. (2002) 'War on the third world'. *The Guardian*, 5 March 2002, p. 15.

Moodley, P. (1995) 'Reaching Out', in S. Fernando (ed.) *Mental Health in a Multi-ethnic Society. A Multi-disciplinary Handbook*. London: Routledge, pp. 120–38.

—— (2002) 'Building a culturally capable workforce – an educational approach to delivering equitable mental health services'. *Psychiatric Bulletin* 26: 63–5.

Morel, B.-A. (1852) *Traite des Mentales*. Paris: Masson (cited by Gottesman, 1991).

Morrison, T. (1993) *Playing in the Dark. Whiteness and the Literary Imagination*. London: Picador (originally published in 1992 by Harvard University Press, Cambridge, MA).

Mukherjee, S., Shukla, S., Woodle, J., Rosen, A. M. and Olarte, S. (1983) 'Misdiagnosis of schizophrenia in bipolar patients: a multiethnic comparison'. *American Journal of Psychiatry* 140: 1571–4.

Murphy, H. B. M. (1973) 'Current trends in transcultural psychiatry'. *Proceedings of the Royal Society of Medicine* 66: 711–16.

Neighbors, H. W., Jackson, J. S., Campbell, L. and Williams, D. R. (1989) 'The influences of racial factors on psychiatric diagnosis: a review and suggestions of research'. *Community Mental Health Journal* 25: 301–11.

Nicholls, V. (2001) *Doing Research Ourselves. A Report of the Strategies for Living Research Support Project.* London: Mental Health Foundation.

Nichter, M. (1980) 'The layperson's perception of medicine as perspective into the utilization of multiple therapy systems in the Indian context'. *Social Science and Medicine* 14B: 225–33.

Nobles, W. W. (1986) 'Ancient Egyptian thought and the development of African (black) psychology', in M. Karenga and J. H. Carruthers (eds) *Kemet and the African World View. Research Rescue and Restoration.* Los Angeles: University of Sankore Press, pp. 100–18.

North East Thames Regional Health Authority and South East Thames Regional Health Authority (1994) *The Report of the Inquiry into the Care and Treatment of Christopher Clunis.* London: HMSO (chairman: J. H. Ritchie).

Obeyesekere, G. (1977) 'Theory and practice of psychological medicine in the Ayurvedic tradition'. *Culture, Medicine and Psychiatry* 1: 155–81.

—— (1985) 'Depression, Buddhism, and the work of culture in Sri Lanka', in A. Kleinman and B. Good (eds) *Culture and Depression.* Berkeley: University of California Press, pp. 134–52.

O'Callaghan, E., Sham, P., Takei, N., Glover, G. and Murray, R. M. (1991) 'Schizophrenia after prenatal exposure to 1957 A2 influenza epidemic'. *Lancet* 337: 1248–50.

Okasha, A. and Ashour, A. (1981) 'Psycho-demographic study of anxiety in Egypt: the PSE in its Arabic version'. *British Journal of Psychiatry* 139: 70–3.

Oldham Independent Panel (2001) *Oldham Independent Review. One Oldham One Future.* Oldham, Greater Manchester: Oldham Metropolitan Borough Council (panel chairman: D. Ritchie).

Omi, M. and Winant, H. (1994) 'Racial formation', in M. Omi and H. Winant (eds) *Racial Formation in the United States: From the Sixties to the Nineties* 2nd edn. New York and London: Routledge, pp. 53–76 (reprinted in P. Essed and D. T. Godlberg (eds) *Race Critical Theories.* Malden, MA and Oxford: Blackwell (2002), pp. 123–45).

Orley, J. and Wing, J. (1979) 'Psychiatric disorders in two African villages'. *Archives of General Psychiatry* 36: 513–20.

Palmer, S. and Laungani, P (1999) *Counselling in a Multicultural Society.* London: Sage.

Pande, G. C. (1995) 'The message of Gotama Buddha and its earliest interpretations', in T. Yoshinori (ed.) *Buddhist Spirituality.* Delhi: Motilal Banarsidass, pp. 3–33.

Parker, S. (1960) 'The Wiitiko psychosis in the context of Ojibwa personality and culture'. *American Anthropology* 62: 603–23.

Parkman, S., Davies, S., Leese, M., Phelan, M. and Thornicroft, G. (1997) 'Ethnic differences in satisfaction with mental health services among representative people with psychosis in South London: PriSM study 4'. *British Journal of Psychiatry* 171: 260–4.

Parveen, T. (1995) 'Services for black communities in general', in C. Harding (ed.) *Not Just Black and White*. An information pack about mental health services for people from Black communities. London: Good Practices in Mental Health, booklet 1.

Pasamanick, B. (1963) 'Some misconceptions concerning differences in the racial prevalence of mental disease'. *American Journal of Orthopsychiatry* 33: 72–86.

Patel, N. (1999) *Getting the Evidence*. London: Mind Publications.

Patterson, O. (1982) *Slavery and Social Death. A Comparative Study*. Cambridge, MA: Harvard University Press.

Pearsall, J. and Trumble, B. (1995) *The Oxford English Reference Dictionary*. Oxford and New York: Oxford University Press.

Pearson, K. (1901) *National Life from the Standpoint of Science*. London: Adam & Charles Black, cited by Fryer, 1984.

Pederson, P. (1998) 'Client-centred interventions as a fourth dimension of psychology', in P. Pederson (ed.) *Multiculturalism as a Fourth Dimension*. London: Mazel, pp. 3–18.

Performance and Innovation Unit (2001) *Scoping note. Improving labour market achievements for ethnic minorities in British society*. http://www.cabinet-office.gov.uk/innovation/test/scope.html

Personal Communication (1996) 'Re C/271/96'. *Letter to S. Fernando from T. Fahy* dated 1 April 1996.

Phillips, T. (2001) 'White flight is enforcing segregation'. *The Guardian*, 19 December 2001, p. 20.

Pick, D. (1989) *Faces of Degeneration. A European Disorder, c. 1848–c. 1918*. Cambridge: Cambridge University Press.

Pieterse, J. N. (1991) 'Fictions of Europe'. *Race and Class* 32(3): 3–10.

Porter, R. (1990) *Mind-forged Manacles. A History of Madness in England from the Restoration to the Regency*. Harmondsworth: Penguin Books (first published by Athlone Press, London 1987).

—— (2002) *Madness. A Brief History*. Oxford: Oxford University Press.

Prabhavandanda, S. and Isherwood, C. (trans.) (1947) *The Song of God. Bhagavad Gita*. London: Phoenix House.

Prichard, J. C. (1835) *A Treatise on Insanity and Other Disorders Affecting the Mind*. London: Sherwood, Gilbert and Piper.

Prince, R. (1968) 'The changing picture of depressive syndromes in Africa'. *Canadian Journal of African Studies* 1: 177–92.

Quraishy, B. and O'Connor, T. (1991) 'Denmark: no racism by definition'. *Race and Class* 32(3): 114–19.

Rack, P. (1982) *Race, Culture and Mental Disorder*. London: Tavistock.

Räthzel, N. (1991) 'Germany: one race, one nation?' *Race and Class* 32(3): 31–48.

Ratnavale, D. N. (1973) 'Psychiatry in Shanghai, China: observations in 1973'. *American Journal of Psychiatry* 130: 1082–7.

Rawnsley, K. (1987) *Face the Facts*. Radio 3, BBC, 23 November 1987.

Richards, D. (1985) 'The implications of African-American spirituality', in M. K. Asante and K. W. Asante (eds) *African Culture: The Rhythms of Unity*. Wesport, CT: Greenwood Press, pp. 207–31.

Richards, G. (1997) *'Race', Racism and Psychology. Towards a Reflexive History*. London: Routledge.

Rogers, J. A. (1942) *Sex and Race. A History of White, Negro, and Indian Miscegenation in the Two Americas* vol. 2. St Petersburg, FL: Helga M. Rogers.

Rosen, G. (1968) *Madness in Society*. New York: Harper & Row.

Rosenthal, D. and Frank, J. D. (1958) 'The fate of psychiatric clinic outpatients assigned to psychotherapy'. *Journal of Nervous and Mental Disease* 127: 330–43.

Ross, R. (1992) *Dancing with a Ghost. Exploring Indian Reality*. Markham, Ontario: Reed Books.

Rumbaut, R. D. (1972) 'The first psychiatric hospital in the western world'. *American Journal of Psychiatry* 128: 125–9.

Ryle, A. (1963) *The Concept of Mind*. Harmondsworth: Penguin.

Sachs, L. (1989) 'Misunderstanding as therapy: doctors, patients and medicines in a rural clinic in Sri Lanka'. *Culture, Medicine and Psychiatry* 13: 335–49.

Said, E. W. (1994) *Culture and Imperialism*. London: Vintage.

St Clair, H. R. (1951) 'Psychiatry interview experiences with Negroes'. *American Journal of Psychiatry* 108: 113–19.

Salman, R. Tuner, S. and Lessing, A. (eds) (1999) *Handbuch interkulturelle Suchthilfe. Modelle, Konzepte und Ansätze der Prävention, Beratung und Therapie*. Gießen: Psychosozial-Verlag.

Sandor, A. (2001) 'Home treatment service'. *Psychiatric Bulletin* 25: 486–7.

Sarbin, T. R. and Mancuso, J. C. (1980) *Schizophrenia: Medical Diagnosis or Moral Verdict?* New York: Pergamon.

Sashidharan, S. P. (2001) 'Institutional racism in British psychiatry'. *Psychiatric Bulletin* 25: 244–7.

Sassoon, M. and Lindow, V. (1995) 'Consulting and empowering black mental health system users', in S. Fernando (ed.) *Mental Health in a Multi-ethnic Society. A Multi-disciplinary Handbook*. London: Routledge, pp. 89–106.

Sayce, L. (2000) *From Psychiatric Patient to Citizen*. London: Macmillan.

Scheff, Thomas J. (1966) *Being Mentally Ill: a Sociological Theory*. Chicago: Aldine.

Schneider, K. (1959) *Clinical Psychopathology*. New York: Grune and Stratton.

Scott, R. D. (1960) 'A family-orientated psychiatric service to the London borough of Barnet'. *Health Trends* 12: 65–8.

Scull, A. (1977) *Decarceration. Community Treatment and the Deviant. A Radical View*. Englewood Cliffs, NJ: Prentice Hall (reprinted as second edition by Polity Press, Cambridge, 1984).

Selten, J. P., and Slaets, J. P. J. (1994) 'Evidence against maternal influenza as a risk factor for schizophrenia'. *British Journal of Psychiatry* 164: 674–6.

——, Slaets, J. P. J. and Kahn, R. S. (1997) 'Schizophrenia in Surinamese and Dutch Antillean immigrants to The Netherlands: evidence of an increased incidence'. *Psychological Medicine* 27: 807–11.

Shallice, A. and Gordon, P. (1990) *Black People, White Justice? Race and the Criminal Justice System*. London: Runnymede Trust.

Shoenberg, E. (ed.) (1972) *A Hospital Looks at Itself*. Plymouth: Cassirer.

Simon, B. and Weiner, H. (1966) 'Models of mind and mental illness in ancient Greece'. *Journal of the History of the Behavioural Sciences* 2: 303–14.

Simon, R. I. (1965) 'Involutional psychosis in Negroes'. *Archives of General Psychiatry* 13: 148–54.

Simon, R. J., Fleiss, J. L., Gurland, B. J., Stiller, P. R. and Sharpe, L. (1973) 'Depression and schizophrenia in hospitalised black and white mental patients'. *Archives of General Psychiatry* 28: 509–12.

Simons, R. C. and Hughes, C. C. (eds) (1985) *The Culture-bound Syndromes. Folk Illnesses of Psychiatric and Anthropological Interest*. Dordrecht: Reidel.

Singh, G. (2001) 'Interview by Emma Brockes'. *The Guardian* G2 Section, 31 December 2001, p. 9.

Singh, R. (1975) 'Depression in ancient Indian literature'. *Indian Journal of Psychiatry* 17: 148–53.

Sivanandan, A. (1985) 'RAT and the degradation of black struggle'. *Race and Class* 26: 1–33.

—— (ed.) (1991) 'Europe. Variations on a theme of racism'. *Race and Class* 32: 3.

Solomos, J., Findlay, B., Jones, S., and Gilroy, P. (1982) 'The organic crisis of British capitalism and race: the experience of the seventies', in Centre for Contemporary Studies (ed.) *The Empire Strikes Back. Race and Racism in 70s Britain*. London: Hutchinson, pp. 9–46.

Special Hospitals Service Authority (SHSA) (1993) *Report of the Committee of Inquiry into the Death in Broadmoor Hospital of Orville Blackwood and a Review of the Deaths of Two Other Afro-Caribbean Patients: 'Big, Black and Dangerous?'* London: Special Hospitals Service Authority (chairman: Professor H. Prins).

Stone, A., Pinderhughes, C., Spurlock, J. and Weinberg, M. D. (1979) 'Report of the committee to visit South Africa'. *American Journal of Psychiatry* 136: 1498–1506.

Strakowski, S. M., Hawkins, J. M., Keck, P. E., *et al.* (1997) 'The effects of race and information variance on disagreement between psychiatric emergency service and research diagnosis in first-episode psychosis'. *Journal of Clinical Psychiatry* 58: 457–63.

——, Lonczak, H. S., Sax, K., West, S. A., Crist, A., Mehta, R. and Thienhaus, O. J. (1995) 'The effects of ethnicity on diagnosis and disposition from a psychiatric emergency service'. *Journal of Clinical Psychiatry* 56: 101–7.

——, Shelton, R. K. and Kolbrener, M. (1993) 'The effects of race and comorbidity on clinical diagnosis in patients with psychosis'. *Journal of Clinical Psychiatry* 54: 96–102.

Strecker, E. A. and Ebaugh, F. G. (1931) *Practical Clinical Psychiatry for Students and Practitioners* 3rd edn. Philadelphia: Blackiston's.

Stubbs, P. (1993) '"Ethnically sensitive" or "anti-racist"? Models for health research and service delivery', in W. I. U. Ahmad (ed.) *'Race' and Health in Contemporary Britain*. Buckingham: Open University Press, pp. 34–47.

Summerfield, D. (2001) 'Does psychiatry stigmatise?' *Journal of the Royal Society of Medicine* 94: 148–9.

Susruta (1963) *Susruta Samhita* (K. S. Bhisagratne ed. and trans.). Varanasi, India: Chowkainbra Sanskrit Series Office.

Susser, E., Lin, S. P., Brown, A. S., Lumey, L. H. and Erlenmeyer-Kimling, L. (1994) 'No relation between risk of schizophrenia and prenatal exposure to influenza in Holland'. *American Journal of Psychiatry* 151: 922–4.

Swartz, L., Ben-Arie, O. and Teggin, A. F. (1985) 'Subcultural delusions and hallucinations. Comments on the Present State Examination in a multi-cultural context'. *British Journal of Psychiatry* 146: 391–4.

Szasz, Thomas S. (1962) *The Myth of Mental Illness*. London: Secker and Warburg.

Thomas, A. and Sillen, S. (1972) *Racism and Psychiatry*. New York: Brunner/Mazel.

Thomas, P. (1997) *The Dialectics of Schizophrenia*. London: Free Association Books.

Tilby, A. (1989) 'Personality clash'. *The Listener*, 16 March 1989, pp. 10–11.

Torrey, E. F. (1973) 'Is schizophrenia universal? An open question'. *Schizophrenia Bulletin* 7: 53–7.

——, Rawlings, R. and Waldman, I. N. (1988) 'Schizophrenic births and viral disease in two states'. *Schizophrenia Research* 1: 73–7.

Toynbee, P. (2001) 'Religion must be removed from all functions of state'. *The Guardian*, 12 December 2001, p. 18.

Tribe, R and Raval, H. (2003) *Working with Interpreters in Mental Health*. East Sussex: Brunner-Routledge.

Trierweiler, S. J., Neighbors, H. W., Munday, C., Thompson, E. E., Binion, V. J. and Gomez, J. P. (2000) 'Clinician attributions associated with the diagnosis of schizophrenia in African American and non-African American patients'. *Journal of Consulting and Clinical Psychology* 68(1): 171–5.

Tuke, D. H. (1858) 'Does civilization favour the generation of mental disease?' *Journal of Mental Science* 4: 94–110.

Turbot, J. (1996) 'Religion, spirituality and psychiatry: conceptual, cultural and personal challenges'. *Australian and New Zealand Journal of Psychiatry* 30: 720–7.

Turkle, S. (1980) 'French anti-psychiatry', in D. Ingleby (ed.) *Critical Psychiatry. The Politics of Mental Health*. New York: Pantheon Books, pp. 150–83.

Unwin, L. (2001) 'Career progression and job satisfaction. Is the selection process for becoming a consultant racist?' in N. Coker (ed.) *Racism in Medicine. An Agenda for Change*. London: King's Fund, pp. 121–38.

Van Praag, H. M. (1976) 'About the impossible concept of schizophrenia'. *Comprehensive Psychiatry* 17(4): 481–97.

Veith, I. (1966) (trans.) *The Yellow Emperor's Classic of Internal Medicine*. Berkeley, LA: University of California Press.

Virdee, S. (1997) 'Racial harassment', in T. Modood, R. Berthoud, J. Lakey, P. Smith, V. Satnam and S. Beishon (eds) *Ethnic Minorities in Britain. Diversity and Disadvantage*. London: Policy Studies Institute, pp. 259–89.

Walvin, J. (1993) *Black Ivory*. London: Fontana Press.

Warner, R. (1983) 'Recovery from schizophrenia in the third world'. *Psychiatry* 46: 197–212.

Watters, C. (2002) 'Migration and mental health care in Europe: report of a preliminary mapping exercise'. *Journal of Ethnic and Migration Studies* 28(1): 153–72.

Watts, A. W. (1971) *Psychotherapy East and West*. London: Jonathan Cape (originally published by Pantheon Books, New York, 1961).

Watts, F. N. and Bennett, D. H. (1983) *Theory and Practice of Psychiatric Rehabilitation*. Chichester: John Wiley.

Waxler, N. (1974) 'Culture and mental illness'. *Journal of Nervous and Mental Illness* 159(6): 379–95.

—— (1979) 'Is outcome for schizophrenia better in non-industrial societies? The case of Sri Lanka'. *Journal of Nervous and Mental Disease* 167: 144–58.

—— (1984) 'Behavioral convergence and institutional separation: an analysis of plural medicine in Sri Lanka'. *Culture, Medicine and Psychiatry* 8: 187–205.

Webb-Johnson, A. (1991) *A Cry for Change. An Asian Perspective on Developing Quality Mental Health Care*. London: Confederation of Indian Organisations.

Weber, M. M. and Engstrom, E. J. (1997) 'Kraepelin's "diagnostic cards": the confluence of clinical research and preconceived categories'. *History of Psychiatry* 8: 375–85.

Weindling, P. (1989) *Health, Race and German Politics Between National Unification and Nazism*. Cambridge: Cambridge University Press.

Wellman, D. (1977) *Portraits of White Racism*. Cambridge: Cambridge University Press.

Wenham, M. (1993) *Funded to Fail: Nuff Pain No Gain. The Under-resourcing of the African-Caribbean Voluntary Sector in London*. London: African-Caribbean Community Development Unit.

Wessely, S., Castle, D., Der, G. and Murray, R. M. (1991) 'Schizophrenia and Afro-Caribbeans. A case-control study'. *British Journal of Psychiatry* 159: 795–801.

West, C. (1994) *Race Matters*. New York: Random House.

Whaley, A. (2001) 'Cultural mistrust of white mental health clinicians among African Americans with severe mental illness'. *American Journal of Orthopsychiatry*, 71(2): 252–6.

Wilson, D. C. and Lantz, E. M. (1957) 'The effect of culture change on the Negro race in Virginia, as indicated by a study of state hospital admissions'. *American Journal of Psychiatry* 114: 25–32.

Wing, J. K. (1978) *Reasoning about Madness*. Oxford: Oxford University Press.

—— (1985) 'The PSE in different cultures'. *British Journal of Psychiatry* 147: 325–6.

—— (1989) 'Schizophrenic psychoses: causal factors and risks', in P. Williams, G. Wilkinson and K. Rawnsley (eds) *The Scope of Epidemiological Psychiatry*. London: Routledge, pp. 225–39.

——, Cooper, J. E. and Sartorius, N. (1974) *Measurement and Classification of Psychiatric Symptoms*. London: Cambridge University Press.

—— and Haley, A. M. (1972) *Evaluating a Community Psychiatric Service*. London: Oxford University Press.

World Health Organisation (1973) *Report of the International Pilot Study of Schizophrenia* vol. 1. Geneva: World Health Organisation.

—— (1979) *Schizophrenia: an International Follow-up Study*. London: Wiley.

Yamamoto, J., James, Q. C., Bloombaum, M. and Hattem, J. (1967) 'Racial factors in patient selection'. *American Journal of Psychiatry* 124: 630–6.

Yamamoto, J., James, Q. C. and Palley, N. (1968) 'Cultural problems in psychiatric therapy'. *Archives of General Psychiatry* 19: 45–9.

Yoshinori, T. (ed.) (1995) 'Introduction', in T. Yoshinori (ed.) *Buddhist Spirituality*. Delhi: Motilal Banarsidass, pp. xiii–xxvi.

Younge, G. (2002) 'Britain is again white'. *The Guardian*, 18 February 2002, p. 13.

Youssef, H. A. and Youssef, F. A. (1996) 'Evidence for the existence of schizophrenia in medieval Islamic society'. *History of Psychiatry* 7: 55–62.

Zilborg, G. (1941) *A History of Medical Psychology*. New York: Norton.

Index